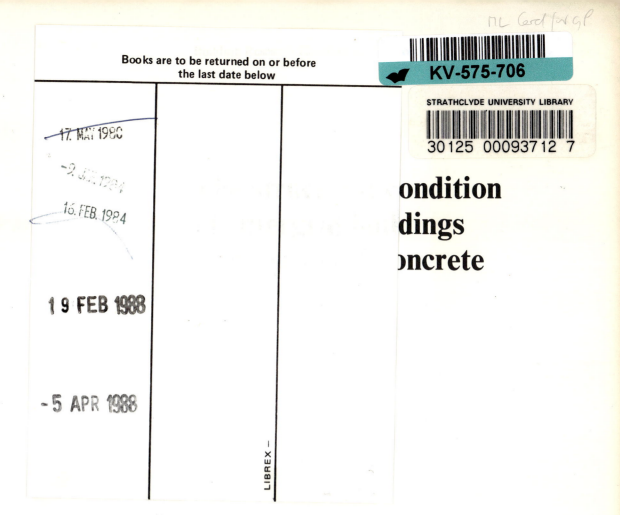

ondition
dings
oncrete

Department of the Environment
Building Research Establishment

London, Her Majesty's Stationery Office

Full details of all new BRE publications
are published quarterly in BRE NEWS.
Requests for BRE NEWS or placing on
the mailing list should be addressed to:
Distribution Unit
Application Services Division
Building Research Station
Garston, Watford WD2 7JR

ISBN 0 11 670753 4
© Crown copyright 1978
First published 1978

Contents

Note: In this report the chloride content of concrete is expressed in terms of the percentage of chloride ion by weight of the cement except where quotations are given which express them in a different form. To convert to chloride content expressed as a percentage of equivalent anhydrous calcium chloride by weight of cement the percentage chloride ion content should be multiplied by 1.565.

For the purposes of this report, high, medium and low chloride contents of concrete are defined as more than 1.0%, between 0.4% and 1.0%, and not exceeding 0.4% chloride ion by weight of cement respectively. The corresponding values in terms of equivalent anhydrous calcium chloride by weight of cement are more than 1.5%, between 0.6% and 1.5% and not exceeding 0.6% respectively.

Summary

Following the discovery in October 1976 of deterioration of pretensioned Intergrid columns caused by corrosion of steel tendons associated with high chloride content in the precast concrete in a school building, the Building Research Establishment extended its field and laboratory investigations of corrosion of steel embedded in concrete. The purpose of the extended investigations which included an analysis of reports of inspections undertaken by owners, was to determine the condition of Intergrid structures and the amount and distribution of chloride in the prestressed concrete Intergrid building components and to provide information relevant to maintaining each Intergrid building in a safe and serviceable condition in the future. Such information would be concerned with the factors affecting tendon corrosion and its detection, techniques of inspection and testing and relationships to the type of structure and structural safety.

From the reports of the inspections at the majority of the 171 Intergrid sites which comprised more than 200 contracts, the prestressed structures appeared to be in good condition. The reported incidence of visible defects associated with corrosion of the embedded steel was low. Earlier tendon fractures had been found in 1974 in one beam which had collapsed after 12 years in service in a non standard Intergrid building and, in these investigations, in one seriously cracked pretensioned column corrosion was found to have caused a break in one tendon after 20 years in service. Visible cracking, spalling or rust staining of the concrete associated with corrosion of tendons or secondary reinforcement was found in about a quarter of column components at two sites and in a few beams at 16 sites and a few columns at 17 sites. Surface corrosion of external tendons of post-tensioned beams was reported by owners' engineers at four sites. It was observed during Building Research Establishment inspections at five other sites and had progressed in the kitchen and shower areas at one site producing significant loss of cross-section. Locations were found in externally-stressed post-tensioned beams where the tendons are more susceptible to corrosion.

Chemical tests on concrete samples indicated that the components in more than two-thirds of buildings for which results were available, ie at 109 sites, have low chloride contents (not exceeding 0.4% chloride ion by weight of cement). Two or more samples from beams in 25 contracts were found to contain at least medium chloride content (between 0.4% and 1.0% chloride ion by weight of cement) and, for columns, 13 contracts yielded two or more samples with at least medium chloride content. Generally these components were manufactured before 1964. Positive indication that calcium chloride was used in the manufacture of components was given in the reported results from beams in nine contracts and from columns in five contracts. Four manufacturers are believed from the evidence to have produced some of these components; the manufacturers of the remainder could not be identified.

Information from the field and laboratory investigations and from experience elsewhere indicated that the time scale associated with corrosion of tendons in any prestressed concrete component in service cannot be predicted accurately. In extreme cases severe corrosion of tendons in exposed columns of the most seriously affected structures had occurred within 20 years; severe corrosion of tendons in a post-tensioned beam indoors, but in a duct partly filled with water, occurred after only 12 years. Tendon corrosion was found to commence locally usually resulting in a substantial loss of cross-section before the full length became affected.

The risk and the time scale of corrosion of the embedded steel is determined by the joint action of several factors. Chloride content of the concrete, age, reduction in alkalinity in the vicinity of the steel associated with permeability and carbonation of the concrete and exposure to moisture were the major factors. Consequently it is not possible to identify a level of chloride content below which corrosion of tendons in prestressed concrete will not occur in the normally expected building life of, say, 50 years since the action of other factors alone may lead to corrosion and present experience extends over only 23 years for Intergrid structures. However the risk of progressive corrosion may become significant above 0.4% chloride ion by weight of cement within the expected life of the structure in circumstances where the steel is in an alkaline environment and the concrete exposed to moisture. Indoors the risk appears to be much less than for external exposure except for components in damp locations, eg where there is roof leakage or heavy condensation.

Most Intergrid structures appear to be insensitive to extensive collapse following failure of one component. The sensitivity to extensive collapse is dependent on the structural design and will be increased if groups of adjacent beam or column components become weakened in the course of time by corrosion of tendons. The safety of roofs in Intergrid buildings is more likely to be adversely affected by tendon corrosion than that of floors.

The BRE investigation showed that, once chloride levels have been established, periodical inspection by an experienced engineer is the best available means of establishing the significance of any deterioration in the condition of the structures.

List of figures

List of plates

1 Introduction

In October 1976 deterioration of pretensioned concrete columns in a building was drawn to the attention of the Building Research Establishment by a consulting engineer. It had been observed during a structural inspection of a school which had been built using the Intergrid system of construction about 20 years previously. The Building Research Establishment took part in investigation of the deterioration which was found to be due to corrosion of the steel tendons associated primarily with the presence of high chloride content in the concrete probably arising from the use of calcium chloride as an accelerator during manufacture of the components.

Previously, in May 1974, a 12 year old post-tensioned concrete roof beam in a non standard Intergrid commercial building had collapsed without warning (see Section 7). After the collapse, several buildings for which components were made by the same manufacturer were identified. The owners, who were public authorities, were advised to inspect them but no adverse reports on their condition were received. The roof beams in one of these buildings which were inspected by the Building Research Establishment were found to have low chloride contents and no apparent signs of corrosion. The collapse was therefore considered to be an isolated incident and no further action was taken at that time.

Corrosion of reinforcement in reinforced concrete leads to visible cracking and spalling of the concrete accompanied by rust-staining of the concrete surface before a serious loss of structural capacity occurs. Similar signs may not appear in prestressed concrete before fracture of the tendons and failure of the component since the tendons are generally of smaller diameter than reinforcement and are more highly stressed.

In view of the implications for public safety of deterioration observed in the Intergrid buildings wider investigations were started by the Building Research Establishment in 1976 at the request of the Departments of the Environment and of Education and Science. The investigation extended a continuing programme of research at the Establishment into the effects of chlorides in concrete on the susceptibility of embedded steel to corrosion.

The Department of Education and Science issued a letter in December 1976 to owners of similar school buildings where the columns were thought to have come from the same source advising that the columns in these schools should be visually inspected as a first stage in dealing with the problem.[1] The inspections identified more buildings with deteriorated columns associated with the presence of high chloride content in the concrete. Consequently, the Department of Education and Science and the Department of the Environment issued letters in March 1977 to owners of all Intergrid buildings which had been identified with the assistance of the proprietors of the system, Gilbert Ash Limited.[2]

The letters, which were prepared with the support of Gilbert Ash Limited and their consulting engineers, Messrs Lowe and Rodin, informed owners of the defects which had been found and of the view of the consulting engineers that, since the use of additives was forbidden in their specifications, they did not believe that many components in Intergrid buildings contained significant amounts of calcium chloride. However, since the possibility could not be excluded that calcium chloride might be present in individual buildings, the letters advised owners of the consulting engineer's view that prestressed columns and pretensioned and post-tensioned prestressed roof and floor beams in Intergrid buildings should be visually inspected and that the concrete should be screened by chemically testing samples for the presence of chloride. Advice on inspection and testing which had been prepared in consultation with the Building Research Establishment was provided (Appendix A). It was suggested that the quality and chloride content of the concrete could be assessed by testing samples taken from 10% of beams and columns from each storey. The advice included the statement:

> 'It may be assumed that calcium chloride has been added to the concrete if two samples out of those taken show a calcium chloride content of over 0.6% equivalent anhydrous calcium chloride by weight of cement'.

The letters also advised owners on action after inspection and testing. It was suggested that the owner's engineer should advise on measures to safeguard the building and its occupants if cracking, spalling or rust-staining of the concrete, or excessive deflection or broken tendons in roof or floor beams was found or if no visible defects were found but the chemical tests indicated that calcium chloride had been added to the concrete. Owners were requested to report the results of their inspections and testing to the Building Research Establishment to assist the investigation and the preparation of further recommendations.

To assist those undertaking the work of sampling and testing the Building Research Establishment published two Information Sheets in July 1977[3, 4].

1

The BRE investigations comprised:

(1) analysis of the reported results of inspections and testing undertaken by owners.

(2) field investigation of a number of selected Intergrid buildings.

(3) laboratory investigations of components taken from buildings in service (in the event no Intergrid components could be made available but some other prestressed and reinforced concrete components from service were examined).

(4) study of experience of inspection techniques and development of new techniques.

(5) review of related research and experience in the UK and overseas of the corrosive effects of chloride in concrete structures containing embedded steel.

The overall requirement was to investigate the effect of chloride in concrete in Intergrid buildings on their structural safety and durability. The investigation required:

(1) determination of the extent of defects and the amount and distribution of chlorides in precast prestressed concrete Intergrid structures.

(2) determination of the effect of chloride content, building age and environmental conditions on tendon corrosion and its consequences.

(3) structural appraisal of the effects of tendon corrosion.

(4) identification and development of inspection and testing techniques.

The results of the investigations are now reported.

2 Origin of chloride in structural concrete

Chloride salts which are present to some extent in most, if not all, structural concretes, originate from impurities in the mix materials, from high concentrations found in the environment, or from deliberate additions of chloride-bearing admixtures during concrete production. In particular chloride ions may be derived from calcium chloride which has been used as an admixture for many years to accelerate the hardening of concrete. The development of the use of this material and the increasing awareness, as a result of experience of the risk of corrosion of embedded steel is described in Appendix B. The first direct advice given in a British Standard Code of Practice against its use specifically to avoid corrosion in prestressed concrete was included in CP 115: 1959. However prior to this date many engineers had become aware of the corrosion risk and prohibited its use in their specifications. In the Intergrid system the use of all admixtures was prohibited. For example, the 1959 and 1964 Intergrid specifications prepared by the consultants and issued by Gilbert Ash Limited stated:

'The concrete shall be made with cement, fine aggregate, coarse aggregate and water, each and all as specified. No other ingredient of any kind shall be added without the permission in writing of the consulting engineer'.

3 Corrosion of steel embedded in concrete

Corrosion of steel with the formation of rust scale (hydrated iron oxide) takes place spontaneously in the presence of water and oxygen. However this corrosion process is inhibited in alkaline environments in the pH range 10 to 13 by the rapid formation of a thin protective film of iron oxide on the metal surface rendering it passive. Thus, although water and oxygen are normally present in exposed concrete, the high alkalinity developed during the hydration of cement is sufficient to provide a high degree of protection to embedded steel against corrosion. It is only when other factors intervene causing impairment or destruction of the protective film on the steel surface that significant corrosion develops resulting in deterioration of the concrete. The first visible effects of such corrosion may sometimes be brown rust staining on the concrete surface without cracking of the concrete*, but this staining usually follows or accompanies cracking generally parallel to the direction of the embedded steel. This cracking occurs because the iron oxide corrosion product occupies a much greater volume than the metallic iron from which it was formed. In addition to staining, cracking and possibly eventual spalling of the concrete, severe corrosion of embedded steel may also cause a reduction in the strength of the structure resulting from the reduced cross-section and tensile capacity of the steel. This reduction in strength is of course more critical with small diameter prestressing steel tendons than with larger diameter reinforcing bars.

When corrosion of steel occurs in concrete it is the result of an electrochemical process associated with variations in the chemical environment around different areas of the steel in the surrounding concrete or occasionally with differences in metallurgical structure. These variations produce electrical potential differences on the steel surface, giving rise to areas that are anodic and cathodic. The resulting electrolytic cells can in some circumstances lead to the significant flow of electrical current in the steel. In the presence of oxygen and water, corrosion can then occur at the anode, iron passing into solution and subsequently forming a rust scale.

The extent of these electro-chemical reactions, and hence the degree and rate of corrosion of steel in concrete, is governed by many different factors. These factors which influence the corrosion behaviour of steel in concrete have been discussed by Verbeck[5]. They are often closely interrelated, but they can be considered to fall into two categories:

(1) physical and environmental factors associated with the quality and physical structure of the concrete and its exposure conditions, and

(2) chemical factors such as the composition of the steel, composition of cement, alkalinity of concrete and the presence of aggressive chemicals, especially free chloride ions.

These factors and the interrelationships between them which are relevant to the condition of Intergrid buildings are discussed below.

Influence of physical and environmental factors

The provision of a cover of well-compacted, dense concrete of low permeability and sufficient thickness in good contact with the steel is of prime importance in preventing corrosion. The permeability of the concrete to the ingress of water, oxygen, carbon dioxide and chloride is governed by its physical structure which depends upon the ingredients and procedures used in making the concrete, including cement content, water/cement ratio, aggregate size and grading, degree of compaction and curing conditions. In general, the permeability of concrete will be increased the lower the cement content, the higher the initial water/cement ratio, and also by inadequate compaction and by unsatisfactory curing conditions. If for one reason or another the concrete has a high permeability, or if the thickness of cover over steel is small or it becomes cracked, then it is possible for the high alkalinity of the concrete environment immediately adjacent to embedded steel to be lost either by leaching of the lime and alkali hydroxides with water or, more commonly, by reaction of atmospheric carbon dioxide with the hydration products of cement, ie by carbonation. Since the stability of the passivating film initially formed on the steel surface is diminished as the alkalinity of the environment is reduced, any reduction in alkalinity by leaching or carbonation will result in the embedded steel becoming more susceptible to corrosion. Moreover, local differences in permeability causing the penetration of different amounts of water, oxygen and carbon dioxide from place to place in a particular concrete component may produce variations in the

---

*Brown rust staining may also occur from other causes, for example the presence of iron-containing aggregate particles at the surface or reinforcement tying wire.

chemical environment of the steel and allow macro-eletrolytic cells to be set up giving localised or sporadic corrosion. The importance of the concrete cover making good contact with embedded steel has been shown in prestressed concrete pipes containing a calcium chloride admixture where severe corrosion was most often found at the site of large air pockets or voids trapped adjacent to the steel[6]. This effect may be connected with the absence of an initially inhibiting film or of any tendency for the rate of corrosion to be reduced through the stifling action of the corrosion product. Similarly, there is likely to be little such stifling action in high-permeability concrete with numerous and large capillary pores whereas in concrete of low permeability, corrosion will be suppressed because the capillary pores will be much smaller in size and number and thus the rate of diffusion of reactants and reaction products will be much lower and diminished further by the blocking action of any corrosion product formed.

The conditions of exposure of the concrete with respect to humidity and temperature can affect the formation and effect of electrolytic cells necessary for corrosion of embedded steel, as well as influencing the depth and rate of carbonation of concrete by atmospheric carbon dioxide. The presence of moisture in concrete is essential for corrosion, and it appears that the most favourable conditions for the formation of electrolytic cells, and hence greatest corrosion, arise at ambient relative humidities in the region of 70–80%. At higher humidities, or with concrete submerged in water, oxygen diffusion to the surface of the steel is considerably reduced. In addition, the environmental conditions in the concrete tend to become more uniform so that electrical potential differences on the steel surface become diminished. It has often been observed that very little corrosion normally occurs in well-made reinforced concrete kept continuously submerged in water, even in the presence of dissolved oxygen and chloride[7]. In contrast, at relative humidities below about 40% very little, if any, free moisture is present in concrete and the necessary condition, ie free water or an aqueous phase for the existence of electrolytic cells, for corrosion is not provided. The effect of increased temperature of exposure within the range normally found in buildings is mainly to increase slightly the rate of the carbonation and electrochemical reactions and of the corrosion process. If chloride is present in the concrete increased temperatures during curing, particularly steam-curing, or on subsequent storage lead to increased amounts of free chloride in solution and hence to a greater extent of corrosion.

Hence, the conditions of exposure of concrete can play a significant role in relation to the extent of corrosion of embedded steel under unfavourable influences. Other factors being equal, steel in concrete exposed to the weather and intermittent wetting and drying will probably be potentially most susceptible to corrosion, while in the absence of water leakages and heavy condensation, the risk and rate of corrosion will generally be reduced for concrete indoors in a dry environment.

Influence of chemical factors

Different types of normal reinforcing and prestressing steels have been indicated to exhibit much the same behaviour in concrete with respect to their durability and resistance to corrosion[5]. The degree and type of stressing applied to prestressing steels normally used in the UK has been found also to have no significant effect. However the initial surface condition of prestressing and normal reinforcing steels, often in practice wholly or partly covered by surface corrosion before embedment, may have some effect on subsequent corrosion behaviour in concrete. It has recently been shown that pre-rusted steel suffers a greater degree of corrosion than shot blasted material when embedded in identical concrete[8]. Furthermore any millscale remaining on the steel surface can act as a cathodic area on the reinforcing steel and can thus stimulate corrosion of the bare steel surfaces, depending upon the alkalinity of the environment and the presence of oxygen and chloride. It has also been observed in some limited laboratory tests on bare steel and uniformly pre-rusted steel embedded in concrete containing chloride that subsequently the degree of localised corrosion with pitting was greater with the bare steel than with the pre-rusted steel[9].

Whilst there is unlikely to be a significant difference in the rate of corrosion of reinforcing steel and prestressing steel when each is embedded separately in concrete, in prestressed concrete construction the electrical contact between secondary reinforcement and prestressing tendons may result in the corrosion of one influencing the tendency to corrosion of the other. This effect may arise because the composition of the steels will be different. It is probably a small effect but it should be noted that it has not been fully investigated. The tendon would normally be more cathodic than the secondary steel and hence should be less prone to corrosion. The electrochemical effect will be small however and would be diminished by the stressing of the tendon (which would tend to make it more anodic) and may be completely eliminated by local effects such as leaching of the alkalies or carbonation of a locally permeable concrete.

There have been several reported instances from overseas[10, 11] where severe and unusual corrosion in the form of cracking occurred in prestressing steel in extensively carbonated high-alumina cement concrete, owing to the use of quenched and tempered steel which was particularly susceptible to corrosion cracking and to the use of high-alumina cement containing an appreciable amount of sulphide capable of modifying the form of corrosion. As far as is known patented and cold-drawn prestressing steel, which is not normally susceptible to this form of attack, was used exclusively in the construction of Intergrid buildings.

The chemical composition and type of cement present in concrete will influence the extent of corrosion of embedded steel to some degree, particularly when chloride is present since the constituents affect the amount of free chloride available in solution, as discussed later. Differences in the amounts of sodium, potassium, and calcium hydroxides available from different cements may also be relevant in relation to the degree and reserve of alkalinity provided in concrete. The higher this alkalinity, the greater the protection afforded against corrosion of embedded steel. As already mentioned, susceptibility to corrosion is increased if the initial high alkalinity becomes reduced either by leaching or by carbonation as determined mainly by the permeability of the concrete, depth of cover and presence of cracks. This reduction in alkalinity is therefore an important chemical factor tending to advance corrosion.

While high alkalinity is a prime requirement for the protection of steel in concrete its benefits are reduced by the presence of free chloride ions. These have the effect, in sufficient quantity, of destroying the protective passivating film of iron oxide on the steel surface so that corrosion can take place at high alkalinity. Thus, even at pH 12.6 (the pH maintained in saturated calcium hydroxide solution) it has been found that passivity can be destroyed by concentrations of free chloride between 35 mg and 700 mg chloride ion/litre[12, 13, 14]. In concrete, however, additional alkalinity derived from sodium and potassium hydroxides released during hydration of the cement will have a marked influence on the level of chloride causing loss of passivity[14]. Since chloride will react with lime, alumina and ferric oxide components of the cement to produce complex hydrated chloride salts (calcium chloroaluminate, $3CaO.Al_2O_3.CaCl_2.1OH_2O$ or calcium chloroferrite, $3CaO.Fe_2O_3.CaCl_2.1OH_2O$, or related solid solutions containing these compounds), only a small proportion of the total chloride is present in the form of ions in solution in any aqueous phase in concrete. Studies carried out to elucidate the many factors involved in controlling the extent of reaction of calcium chloride with cement in concrete have indicated[6, 9, 15] that a large proportion, perhaps up to 90%, of the calcium chloride added as an admixture may exist in a combined form as complex hydrated salts in ordinary Portland cement concrete at normal temperatures, but there will always be some free chloride remaining in solution in any aqueous phase in contact with the complex hydrated chloride salts present in the concrete.

The various factors affecting the proportion and concentration of free chloride in solution (and hence the extent of corrosion) have been studied by Roberts[9]. Thus, investigations of the reaction of calcium chloride with cement in continuously shaken cement pastes of water/cement ratio 1.5 have shown that the final free chloride concentration of the solution in contact with the hydrated cement increases markedly as the initial amount of added chloride increases and also with increasing temperature in the range 25°C to 90°C. In addition, higher free chloride concentrations arise with sulphate-resisting Portland cement as compared with ordinary Portland cement, owing to the decreased tricalcium aluminate content (or increased Fe_2O_3/Al_2O_3 ratio) of the sulphate-resisting Portland cement. This effect of cement composition has actually been reflected in observations of corrosion behaviour in that it has been found that cements with a high tricalcium aluminate content afford increased protection against corrosion in the presence of chloride[5, 9]. Other factors in cement composition may also influence the proportion of free chloride in solution, and it has been indicated that this proportion will be increased the lower the content of alumina and ferric oxide, or the higher the ratio Fe_2O_3/Al_2O_3, or the higher the content of calcium sulphate setting regulator or of free alkali (sodium and potassium hydroxides)[9]. It is clear, therefore, that cement composition can play an important part in relation to the amount of free chloride present in concrete and thereby influence the degree of corrosion of embedded steel.

It must also be recognised that although the chloride content combined in complex hydrated chloride salts in concrete will not play a direct part in corrosion of embedded steel, these chloride compounds form a reservoir of chloride which will be liberated, readily pass into solution and provide accentuated corrosive conditions if leaching with water occurs in the concrete. Moreover, appreciable carbonation of the concrete by atmospheric carbon dioxide or attack of the concrete by sulphate solutions will result in decomposition of the complex hydrated chloride salts, liberating chloride into solution and aggravating corrosion of embedded steel.

Many laboratory investigations have been made to examine the effect of chloride on the corrosion of steel in concrete. In studies reported before 1970 it was generally concluded that severe corrosion of embedded steel does not occur when a restricted amount of chloride (not exceeding 1.0% chloride ion by weight of cement) is present in well-compacted, dense concrete of low permeability[9, 16–19]. In tests with steel bars embedded at 10 mm cover in Portland cement mortar prisms (aggregate/cement = 2.68 and water/cement = 0.45), and subsequently stored at 20°C and 65% relative humidity and sprayed with water every 14 days, Richartz[15] found no signs of any corrosion at all at ages up to 3 years with calcium chloride additions up to 0.4% chloride ion by weight of cement. Furthermore electrochemical tests have indicated[20, 21] that embedded steel can remain passive in Portland cement concrete containing calcium chloride at a level of 0.26% chloride ion by weight of cement, but this passivity is destroyed or not achieved with 0.51% or more chloride ion by weight of cement and the steel then becomes susceptible to corrosion. Similarly, in other electrochemical tests it was found[22] that polished steel remained passive in Portland cement concrete containing sodium chloride at a level of 0.30% chloride ion by weight of cement, but not so with 0.46%, 0.61% and 1.22% chloride ion by weight of cement, nor with more than 0.15% chloride ion in slag cement concrete. In addition recent results obtained by the Building Research Establishment from reinforced concrete samples exposed to the weather revealed corrosion of steel in concrete containing 1.0% chloride ion by weight of cement. After exposure for five years corrosion sufficient to crack the concrete cover had occurred generally over the steel surface where the steel had 10 mm cover and there were indications of localised pitting attack at 20 mm cover in fully alkaline concrete.

Thus present evidence from research investigations does not clearly identify a level of chloride content below which corrosion of steel will not occur. It suggests that corrosion difficulties are unlikely to occur in ordinary Portland cement concrete containing small amounts of chloride in concrete as might arise from impurities in the concrete ingredients, corresponding to less than about 0.4% chloride ion by weight of cement provided that other unfavourable factors, particularly high permeability and low alkalinity, are not present. However the concretes and mortars used in many of the reported research investigations may differ to some extent from those used in practice since greater variations in the composition of the mix, in the permeability of the hardened concrete and in the distribution of chloride may occur under normal commercial conditions. Thus, other unfavourable factors may be present in building construction and it appears possible that, in these circumstances, even lower chloride contents may have an adverse influence on the long-term durability of embedded steel in concrete. There is a much increased risk of progressive corrosion of embedded steel with quantities of chloride above 0.4% chloride ion by weight of cement and the risk is high when the quantity exceeds about 1.0% chloride ion by weight of cement, particularly in concrete exposed to the weather or intermittent wetting and drying.

Summarising, many physical, chemical and environmental factors influence the protection of steel in concrete to some extent but there are three aspects which have major adverse effects on the long-term susceptibility of embedded steel to corrosion:

(1) reduction in alkalinity in the vicinity of the steel associated with permeability and carbonation of the concrete cover.
(2) exposure of the concrete to the weather or intermittent wetting and drying.
(3) the presence of chloride ions in the concrete.

These effects are less for good quality concrete, ie properly-cured, well-compacted concrete with a low water/cement ratio, in dry conditions.

4 The Intergrid system of construction

The Intergrid system was first developed in 1952 by Gilbert-Ash Limited and the Prestressed Concrete Company Limited in conjunction with the Ministry of Education as part of the programme to introduce new methods and materials to aid the school building programme at a time of shortage of labour and traditional materials. The system was originally based upon the use of light modular precast concrete elements of small cross-section, post-tensioned together to form floor and roof beams supported on precast pretensioned columns. Subsequent developments by Gilbert-Ash Limited and their engineering consultants incorporated larger components and pretensioned floor and roof beams. Occasionally, special one-off structures were marketed as Intergrid or special components were incorporated in otherwise standard construction to meet particular requirements. The development of the system is described in more detail below. In all, more than 200 contracts have been completed at 171 sites.

The Prestressed Concrete Company Limited (later the Prestressed Concrete Associates which then became Messrs Lowe and Rodin) were the specialist consultants responsible for the design and specification covering manufacture and erection. The system was designed in accordance with current or draft Codes of Practice of the day, supplemented by floor, roof and column tests. With one or two exceptions, erection was carried out by Gilbert-Ash Limited. Precast components are thought to have been made by at least 18 manufacturers (including Gilbert-Ash) operating from 24 works. In addition some components were precast on site. Inspection was carried out by Gilbert-Ash's own independent engineering inspectorate in accordance with procedures developed in conjunction with the consultants.

The development of the system

The Intergrid system as its name implies was originally conceived as a precast frame with a horizontal two-way prestressed grid using standard components which could be adapted for a variety of spans and structural configurations.

After the prototype structure was built at Worthing the first generally available system was the Mark II Intergrid system produced in 1954 which was subsequently superseded by Marks III, IV, and V over the following 23-year period. The sequence of

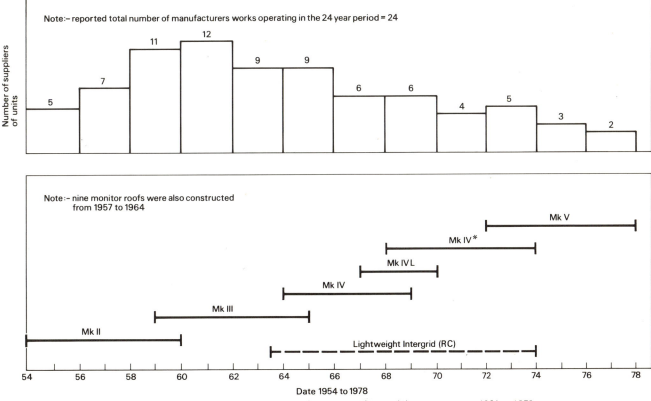

Figure 1 Development of the Intergrid system and numbers of manufacturers works supplying components, 1954 to 1978

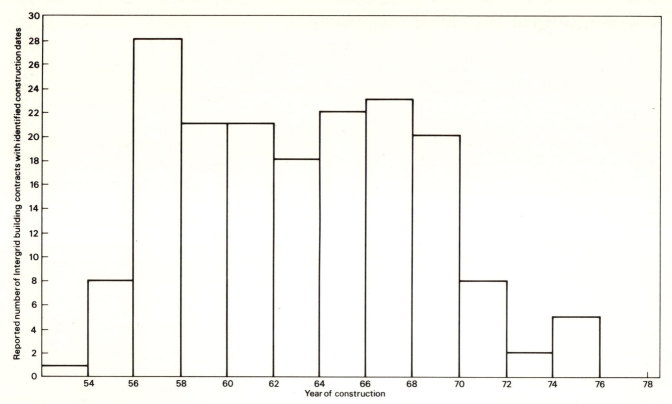

Figure 2 Production of Intergrid from 1954 to 1977

development is given in Figure 1 which also shows the probable numbers of manufacturing works supplying structural components. The distribution of the construction of Intergrid buildings over the 24-year period is indicated in Figure 2.

Generally the structural frame was pin jointed, horizontal stability being provided by vertical bracing panels to which the horizontal forces were transmitted by the floors and roofs. Other than in Mark V roof construction all standard floors and roofs incorporated a secondary load distribution system.

The Mark II system introduced in 1954

The floor and roof beam components comprised of 3′–4″ (1020 mm) precast lattice units as shown in Figure 3. These units were assembled into primary beams by aligning them on the ground using in situ mortar between the units as packing and then stressing them together. The prestress was provided by a number of external post-tensioned 0.200 ins (5 mm) or 0.276 ins (7 mm) diameter wire tendons. In some beams the external tendons were positioned in a longitudinal channel running in the top or sides of the lower flange.

These tendons were hair-pin shaped in plan, the free ends of each tendon being anchored at low level at one end of the beam. The tendons were positioned externally along the top of the lower flange, as indicated in Figure 3 and at the opposite end of the beam they were bent up to pass round the mild steel seating assembly. These hair-pin shaped tendons were provided in one or more alternating pairs.

The assembled primary beams were positioned on the column or edge beam substructure at 3′–4″ (1020 mm) centres and secondary units of the same depth and concrete profile placed transversely between the primary

beams, again at 3′–4″ (1020 mm) or 6′–8″ (2040 mm) centres. These transverse units were then stressed together in a similar way to the primary units using external tendons which passed through the lower flange of the primary beams. After stressing, the tendons were covered with mortar and the finished surface and adjacent concrete was usually given a coating of bitumen paint. This process gave a two-way spanning grillage of lattice beams which was readily adaptable to structural requirements by varying the number of prestressing wires in either or both directions (Figure 4).

Although there were differences of detail in the single units according to their function, eg primary beam, transverse (secondary) beams, roof purlins, floor and roof assemblies, the system is based essentially on the lattice unit shown in Figure 3 with special end units for the tendon anchorages and high level seatings.

The infilling of the beam grid which provided the floor decking was usually achieved using square precast concrete slabs which fitted into notches in the top flange of the beams. The whole assembly was then mortar jointed ready to receive the non-structural finishing screed. The roof structure consisted of woodwool slabs

10

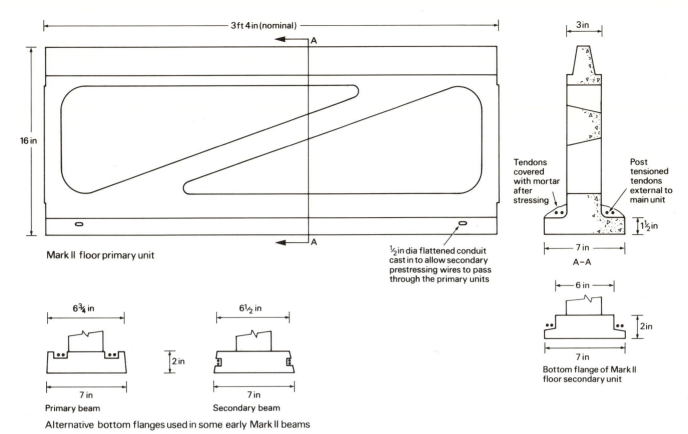

Figure 3 Precast unit for Mark II Intergrid beam

with a reinforced concrete topping which was tied to the beams to form a structurally composite deck.

The columns supporting the Mark II floors and roofs had precast pretensioned shafts to which were bolted separate reinforced concrete head units. The shafts were additionally reinforced with secondary binder reinforcement at the top and bottom of the units. The overall dimensions of cross-section varied slightly according to the type of column but they were generally $6\frac{1}{4}'' \times 4\frac{1}{2}''$ (159 mm × 115 mm) with nibs and recesses provided to accommodate cladding panels and fixings. External columns had at least one face exposed in elevation in the Mark II system. Columns and beams

were mechanically connected using a combination of dowel bar, plates and linked reinforcement which was surrounded with in situ concrete.

Spanning between the column heads were boundary beams; primary or secondary beams were then supported either directly on the column heads or on the boundary beams. The precast boundary beams were of reinforced concrete construction as were the stair landing beams, stair treads and roof lights. The stair rakers however were post-tensioned. According to the requirements of individual clients these Intergrid structures were clad in differing combinations of precast concrete panels, brickwork, timber or tiles.

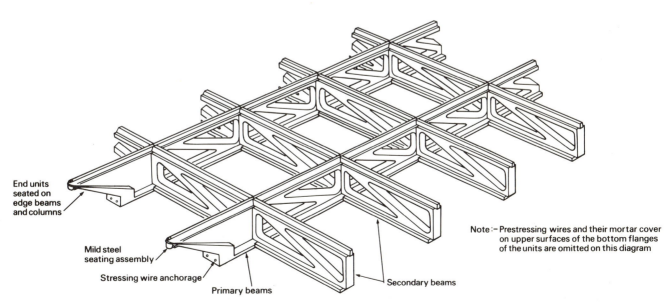

Figure 4 Mark II Intergrid beam grillage (post-tensioned in both primary and secondary directions)

The Mark III system introduced in 1959

The Mark III system was of more conventional construction than the Mark II system. The primary beams were either pretensioned monolithic components or made up of segmental units with internal steel ducts carrying the prestressing tendons which were post-tensioned and grouted on site. Both types of beam had similar profiles and can be regarded as fulfilling the same purpose in the system (Figure 5). Components were available in two section depths, either pretensioned 1′–2½″ (368 mm) or post-tensioned 1′–7½″ (495 mm), the deeper components being used for longer spans or where floor loadings were high. They were generally used at either 3′–4″ (1020 mm), 6′–8″ (2040 mm) or 10′–0″ (3050 mm) centres. Ribbed floor slabs spanned transversely between the primary beams. They were cast in situ on Trafford Tile asbestos sheeting which was used as permanent shuttering. These slabs were stiffened by secondary precast reinforced concrete beams at a maximum of 10′–0″ (3050 mm) centres which were post-tensioned on site (Figure 6).

This form of construction produced a rigid-plate floor stressed in two directions acting compositely with the floor slab as in the Mark II system. However the Mark III system differed from the Mark II in that it had a more clearly defined preferential span direction.

The sequence of floor construction was to position the primary beams on their supports, place the secondary precast units between the primary beams and stress the structure transversely by passing wires through the hollow secondary beams and anchoring them at each end on the structure. The permanent asbestos sheet shuttering was then placed in position and the structural topping cast in situ with the hollow secondary units.

In later Mark III buildings the in situ slab and asbestos sheet shuttering were replaced by 2¾″ or 4¼″ (70 mm or 108 mm) precast floor slabs. Infill concrete over the primary and secondary beams was used to connect the units to form the deck. The rest of the system remained unchanged.

The columns used in conjunction with the Mark III floor had integral heads and were again pretensioned components but of larger cross-section than the Mark II columns. Their overall structural dimensions were 6½″ × 6½″ (165 mm × 165 mm) or 8″ × 8″ (203 mm × 203 mm) with recesses and nibs provided to accommodate cladding details. In a proportion of cases at least one face of the external columns was exposed in elevation. However quite frequently the frame was placed inside the fenestration. The columns were placed usually at either 6′–8″ (2040 mm) or 10′–0″ (3050 mm) centres corresponding to two and three-module bays respectively. Column secondary reinforcement was provided at the top and bottom of the components. This link reinforcement was replaced by helical reinforcement in later Mark III structures.

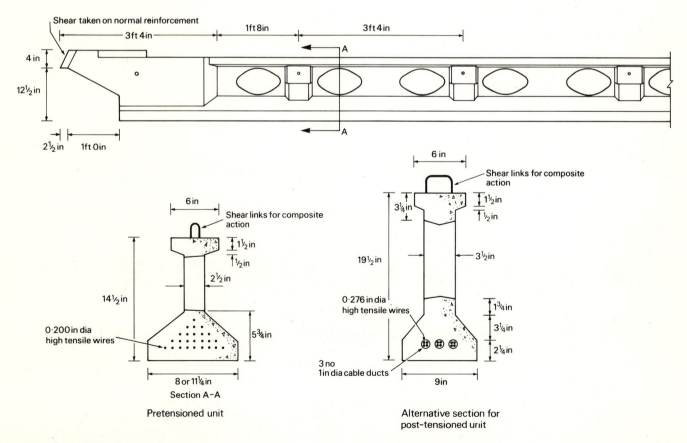

Figure 5 Mark III Intergrid primary beams

12

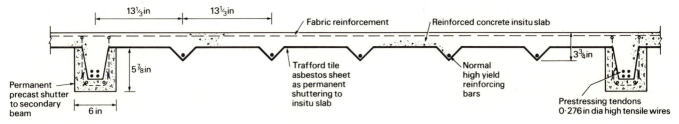

Figure 6 Ribbed floor slab and secondary beam of Mark III Intergrid system

Lightweight Intergrid

Another variation of Intergrid was 'Lightweight Intergrid' which was introduced in 1962. It was not a prestressed system and therefore is strictly outside the scope of this report but it is mentioned here briefly for completeness. 'Lightweight Intergrid' was a single storey load-bearing wall and flat roof system with

isolated concrete beams (Figure 7). The roof deck was normally of Stramit, woodwool or timber boarding. The stability in buildings using this system was provided by cross walls. Where columns were used they were 6½″ × 6½″ (165 mm × 165 mm) in cross-section and of precast reinforced concrete construction.

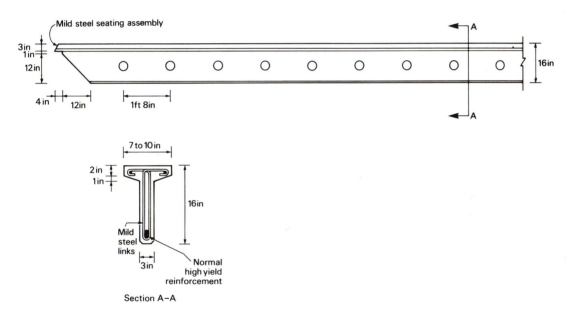

Section A–A

Figure 7 Lightweight Intergrid primary beam

The Mark IV system introduced in 1964

The Mark IV system with its use of bolted secondary beams was a natural development of the Mark III system, as part of the process of reducing the amount of stressing work carried out on site. The only stressing carried out was the post-tensioning of primary roof beams for spans in excess of 40′–0″ (12.2 m).

The primary beams were limited to two types only, one a pretensioned unit 1′–2½″ (368 mm) deep the other a post-tensioned unit in three sections 1′–7½″ (495 mm) deep (Figure 8).

The secondary beams were precast reinforced concrete

units bolted to the primary beams at 3′–4″ (1020 mm) centres in floor construction and generally at 6′–8″ (2040 mm) or 10′–0″ (3050 mm) centres in roof construction (Figure 9).

The structural decking comprised of 2″ (50 mm) thick precast reinforced concrete slabs which were supported on the secondary beams. Additional reinforcement and infill concrete between the floor slabs, over the primary and secondary beams and around the edges was provided to tie the assembly of units together. A 1¼″ (32 mm) thick non-structural floor finishing screed was then laid.

The roof construction used woodwool slabs supported on the primary or secondary beams. The structural topping concrete infilled between the woodwool slabs over the primary and secondary beams and formed a composite deck with a minimum thickness of 1¼″ (32 mm) over the woodwool slabs. This screed was reinforced with a light square fabric mesh and laid to falls of 2″ (50 mm) in 10′–0″ (3050 mm) relative to the mid point of the combined pretensioned primary beams.

The columns were generally the same as those used in the earlier Mark III system being precast prestressed units with structural core dimensions of 6½″ × 6½″ (165 mm × 165 mm) or 8″ × 8″ (203 mm × 203 mm). Load tests were carried out by the consultant on the Mark IV floors to verify their secondary load redistribution characteristics.

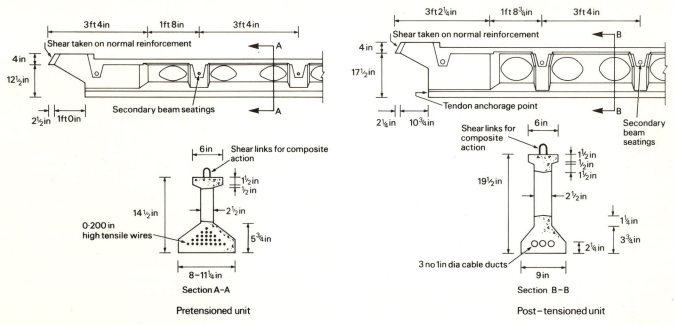

Figure 8 Mark IV Intergrid primary beams

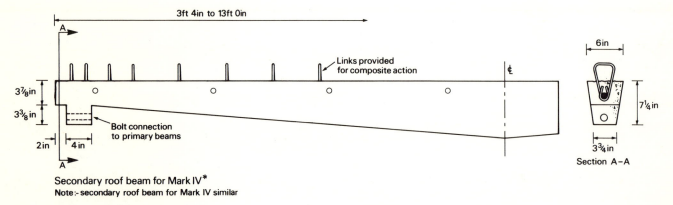

Figure 9 Mark IV Intergrid secondary beam

The Mark IV L system introduced 1966

The horizontal construction in previous Intergrid marks had been based solely on a 3′–4″ module but to meet specific client requirements a 4′–0″ module was designed. It was based on the Mark IV system with the following changes:

(i)   The use of post-tensioned units ceased,

(ii)   A combined secondary beam and floor slab unit was introduced,

(iii) Strand prestressing tendons replaced the 0.200 ins (5 mm) diameter wires in the primary beams, and

(iv)   All the columns were constructed in precast reinforced concrete.

14

The Mark IV* system introduced in 1968

The experience gained from the Mark IVL projects led to an updating of the standard Mark IV (3'–4" module) system.

Items (i) and (ii) and (iii) listed above were taken from the Mark IVL and incorporated to form the new Mark IV* system. The primary beams also underwent some detail changes in profile and stressing (Figure 10). The combined precast floor slab and secondary beam units which spanned between the primary beams were normally reinforced and shaped as shown in Figure 11. The small secondary beams were cast by positioning the floor units next to each other and placing steel in the 'V' shapes formed, then infilling with structural concrete (Figure 12). Shear keys in the floor units were provided to further improve the composite action between the units and the infill concrete, and to help in the transmission of differential load effects between adjacent floor units. The resulting floor construction is much simplified comprising only two basic units with the shuttering all provided by the permanent structural units.

Mark IV* roof construction was generally similar to that used in the Mark IV system.

Pretensioned columns, with only marginal adjustments to the head details remained in use. These had a minimum core dimension of either 6½" (165 mm) or 8" (203 mm), the nibs to receive the cladding being additional to these dimensions. The helical binder steel introduced earlier was retained. Greater emphasis on exfill brickwork cladding often hides these columns from sight.

Mechanical linkages between the columns and beams were provided in the same manner as for the Mark III system using plates, dowels and hooped bars.

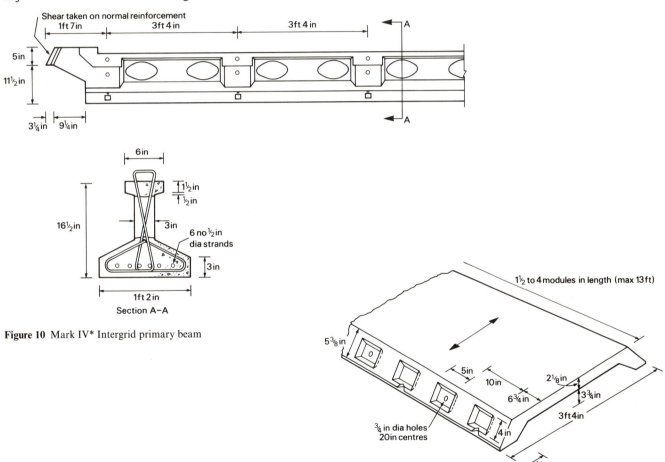

Figure 10 Mark IV* Intergrid primary beam

Figure 11 Mark IV* Intergrid combined floor slab and secondary unit

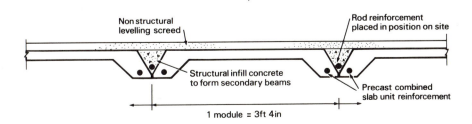

Figure 12 Mark IV* Intergrid combined floor slab and secondary beam assembly

The Mark V system introduced in 1972

The Mark V system is the current metric version of the Intergrid system although metric reinforcement had been used in the Mark IV* system. The original 3'–4" (1020 mm) module was replaced by a 1800 mm module.

The floor system is similar to that used in the Mark IV* system with a few changes in detail. The precast floor primary beams of 7.2 m span and over are pretensioned (Figure 13) whilst the smaller units are of reinforced concrete construction. The combined floor slab units are retained except that they now correspond to the new module sizes. However the roof construction was entirely redesigned using variable depth isolated precast prestressed beams and profiled metal decking. The primary roof beams are 'T' shaped as detailed in Figure 14 and those of 10.8 m span and over are pretensioned using 15.2 mm diameter strand reinforcement, those of smaller span being normally reinforced. The upper surfaces of the beams are cambered in order to build in the necessary drainage falls.

The columns are 250 mm square and constructed in precast reinforced concrete. These are often cast in building height lengths. Beams and columns are normally at 3.6 m centres.

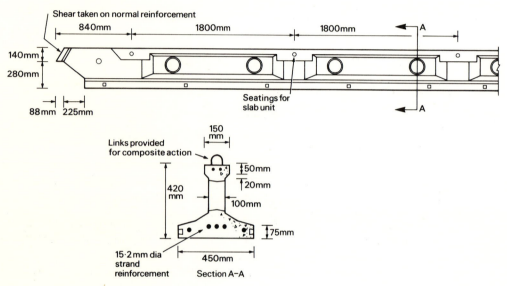

Figure 13 Mark V Intergrid primary floor beam

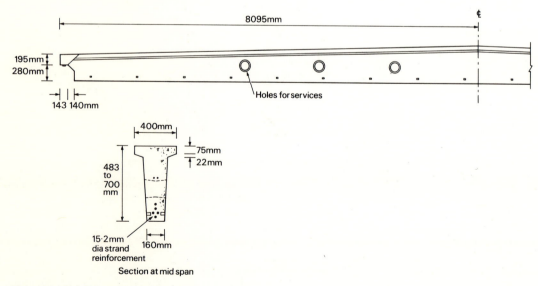

Figure 14 Mark V Intergrid typical primary roof beam

16

Non-standard Intergrid

(i) The monitor system

These roof structures were designed and constructed by the same organisations as the other standard Intergrid systems but can be regarded as totally different in concept. The monitor roof beams were intended primarily for large span single-storey lightweight roof construction. Nine monitor structures were built over the period 1957 to 1964 and although they all had similar concrete profiles their spans ranged from 37 ft (11.1 m) to 80 ft (34.4 m), being assembled from precast units post-tensioned together. An example of an 80 ft (24.4 m) span post-tensioned beam is shown in Figure 15.

Precast normally-reinforced concrete purlins spanned between the monitor beams supporting roofing material which was usually lightweight asbestos or translucent plastic sheeting. The purlins were bolted into the top boom of the monitor beams with through-bolts. The roof structures were made up in effect of a number of isolated long-span beams in which the tie chord is provided by a post-tensioned component.

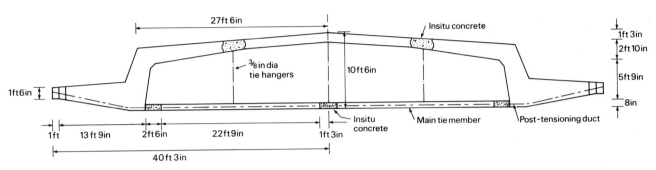

Figure 15 Monitor roof beam

(ii) Other non-standard Intergrid systems

Occasionally special one-off structures were marketed as Intergrid or special components were incorporated into otherwise standard construction to meet particular requirements of increased loading or span.

In addition there are cases in which the primary beams are isolated and not of composite construction, a change which may affect the secondary load distribution characteristic of the structure.

Special roof profiles were also required at times which resulted in the monitor system mentioned above and some 'North-Light' forms of construction.

5 Reports on inspections of Intergrid buildings undertaken by owners

By 31 December 1977 the Building Research Establishment had received reports from 133 sites out of the total of 171 sites identified and 109 of these included information on visual inspection and the results of tests for chloride made on samples of the concrete.

The number of local authorities indicated as owners in the reports was 42 and there were 18 other owners involved. The buildings at the majority of the sites (106) were schools. Office buildings occupied 12 sites and buildings on 15 sites were used for other purposes. Most sites contained more than one Intergrid building and the buildings were sometimes of a different Intergrid Mark constructed in separate building contracts. The numbers of contracts for which reports on buildings of each Intergrid Mark were received are shown in Table 1 and compared with the total number of contracts.

The reports of inspections indicated that most Intergrid buildings had no visible defects associated with corrosion of tendons or reinforcement and that, where visible defects were present, they were confined to a minority of components. There were reports of rust staining on a few beams at 12 sites and at ten of these sites, cracking was also reported. At a further four sites cracking in a few beams was found without any rust staining reported. For pretensioned columns the reported incidence of visible defects was more numerous, two sites having about a quarter of external columns with either rust staining, cracking, or spalling reported and 17 sites having a few columns in a cracked or spalled condition.

The number of samples of concrete taken for chemical analysis varied widely. In many cases the reports contained results from samples taken from fewer than 10% of components. High alumina cement concrete was reported to have been used in the manufacture of beam components in parts of 16 buildings and in the joints between the precast units in Mark II beams. This concrete was not usually sampled.

The reported results of the analyses are shown in Figures 16 and 17 in terms of the number of building contracts from which samples were taken and showing the numbers where two or more samples were found to contain chloride in the ranges of 0.4% to 1.0% and greater than 1.0% chloride ion by weight of cement. It

Table 1 Number of reports received

Intergrid Mark	Number of contracts reported	Total number of contracts	
Prototype	1	1	(1)
2	48	58	(46)
3	37	49	(39)
4	35	40	(18)
4*	14	34	(23)
4L	2	2	(1)
5	7	9	(7)
Monitor	2	9	(6)
Non-standard	2	—	
Unknown	4	—	

Figures in brackets indicate school contracts

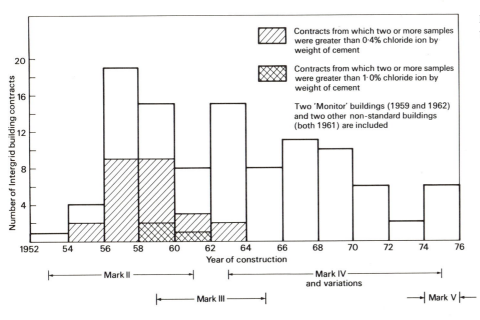

Figure 16 Distribution of contracts from which beam samples were taken

(chart legend)
Contracts from which two or more samples were greater than 0·4% chloride ion by weight of cement

Contracts from which two or more samples were greater than 1·0% chloride ion by weight of cement

Two 'Monitor' buildings (1959 and 1962) and two other non-standard buildings (both 1961) are included

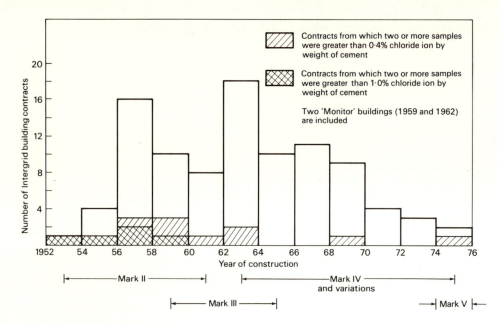

Figure 17 Distribution of contracts from which column samples were taken

can be seen that the components in more than two-thirds of building contracts contain low chloride contents and that where two or more results were greater than 0.4% chloride ion by weight of cement the majority of construction was prior to 1964.

Whilst the levels of chloride content in hardened concrete associated with the addition of calcium chloride in the production of concrete cannot be defined precisely, it was assumed in the Annex to the DOE letter (Appendix A) that, for screening purposes, two or more results above 0.4% chloride ion by weight of cement should be taken as indicating that this admixture was probably used in the manufacture of the beam or column components. This criteria was given to provide a conservative basis for assessing the risk of corrosion to embedded steel but does not provide a positive indication that the admixture was used. It is thought that, bearing in mind the probable errors in reported analyses (Section 9), such indication would be provided only if a representative selection of components were sampled and if a substantial proportion of the samples yielded chloride contents in the medium and high chloride content ranges. In general the greater the proportion of results in these ranges and the higher the results, the more positive is the indication of use of the admixture. In this report it has been assumed that 20 or more similar components should be sampled to provide an adequate number of results and that a positive indication is provided if 20% or more of the results are in the medium or high chloride content ranges or if four or more results are in the high chloride content range.

Applying the criterion in the DOE letter mentioned in the previous paragraph, to the reported results, two or more samples from beams in 25 contracts were found to contain at least medium chloride content and in three of

these contracts two or more samples had high chloride content. For columns, the corresponding figures were 13 contracts yielding two or more samples with at least medium chloride content, five of these contracts giving two or more samples containing high chloride content. Positive indication, as defined above, that calcium chloride was used in the manufacture of the components was given in the reported results from beams in nine contracts and from columns in five contracts.

A summary of the results in terms of the percentages of the total number of analyses reported above 0.4% chloride ion by weight of cement, the date of construction, ie approximate age of components, and the Intergrid Mark is shown in Figures 18 and 19. This confirms that most components contain low chloride contents and that most of those with higher levels of chloride content were found in components manufactured before 1964. It should be noted that the reported results for chloride ion content by weight of cement were not all based on measured cement contents of the samples. The results have been plotted as interpreted in the reports; in some cases an average measured cement content from a proportion of samples was used, in others a cement content of 14% was taken as suggested[2], whilst in others a value of 20% was assumed. These different bases would not markedly affect the overall distributions shown in Figures 18 and 19 but the proportion of results falling above 0.4% chloride ion by weight of cement for an individual building might be substantially changed.

A distribution for the results of tests on concrete samples for chloride content is shown in Figure 20 for columns in a building where calcium chloride was added in manufacture. It can be seen that most results were above the screening limit of 0.4% chloride ion by

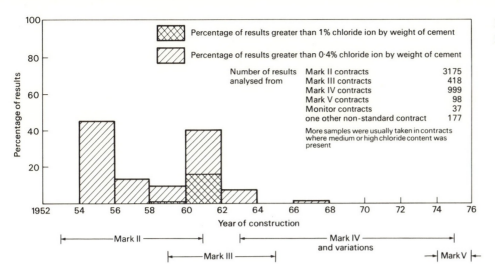

Figure 18 Chloride content in precast prestressed concrete beams

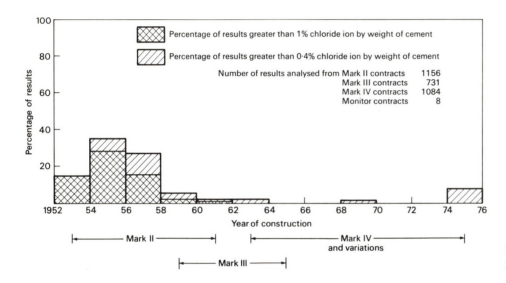

Figure 19 Chloride content in precast prestressed concrete columns

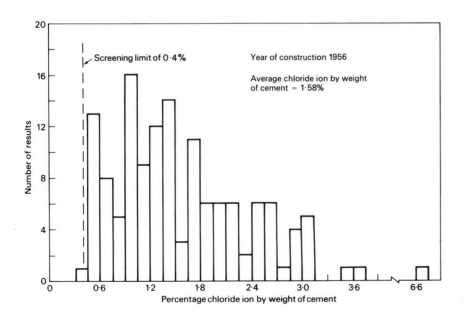

Figure 20 Chloride content of samples from contract 1

weight of cement. In comparison, in Figure 21, a distribution is given for columns supplied by the same manufacturer for the construction of another building. All results were lower than the screening limit and indicate the levels of chloride content which may arise from chlorides occurring naturally in concrete materials. Not all distributions of the reported results from other buildings could be clearly equated with these distributions, significant proportions of their results being above and below the screening limit. These wider distributions with intermediate average values suggested that the samples may have been taken from components taken from two manufacturing batches, from components supplied by different manufacturers or from components where a lower than normal dosage of calcium chloride admixture had been used which had not been thoroughly mixed during manufacture.

Reports on the analyses of samples taken from the mortar cover of tendons in Intergrid Mark II beams were received from 21 sites. In general chloride contents were low (Figure 22). There was no evidence that

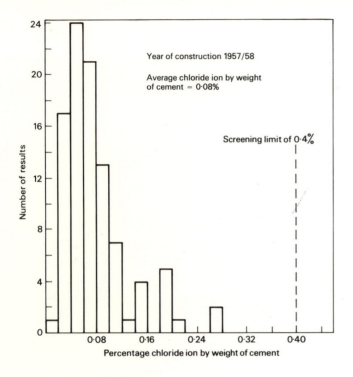

Figure 21 Chloride content of samples from contract 2

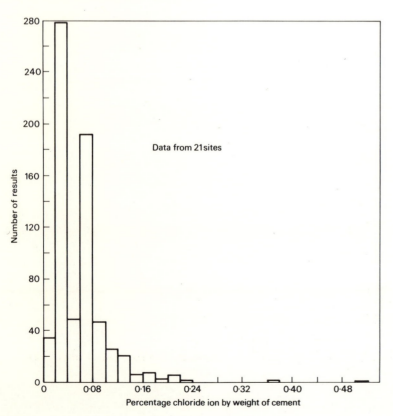

Figure 22 Chloride content of samples from mortar cover of tendons in Mark II beams

22

chlorides had migrated into the mortar from the precast concrete units which in some cases contained medium chloride contents. Cement contents measured on samples of the mortar ranged from 23% to 47% (average 32%). Few reports gave an indication of the degree of compaction or carbonation of the mortar. There was also no indication of the condition of tendons in Mark II beams except from 12 sites where the reported appearance ranged from excellent to satisfactory and from 'clean' to 'slight surface corrosion' to 'slight pitting' and it was concluded that the tendon strength had not been impaired. The findings of BRE investigations of Mark II Intergrid beams are given in Section 7.

The precast concrete itself was reported to be of good quality, cement contents of the concrete samples generally being greater than 14 per cent. Histograms of cement contents for samples taken from beams and columns are shown in Figures 23 and 24 which indicate

the small number of results falling below 14 per cent. Twenty reports contained the results of analyses of samples taken from the in situ OPC mortar or concrete forming the joints between the precast units in beams. These results indicated low chloride contents except in two reports. In one case two out of 12 results showed a medium chloride content and in the other case, seven out of 28 results showed at least medium chloride content, five of these being in the high content range.

Only five reports included mention of carbonation of concrete in Intergrid components. No indication was given of the extent of testing. Tests at one site indicated depth of carbonation in beams of at least 10 mm. None was reported from the other four sites. The results of carbonation tests made by the BRE on Intergrid components are included in Sections 6 and 7.

Water penetration causing wet conditions around some beams was reported at five sites.

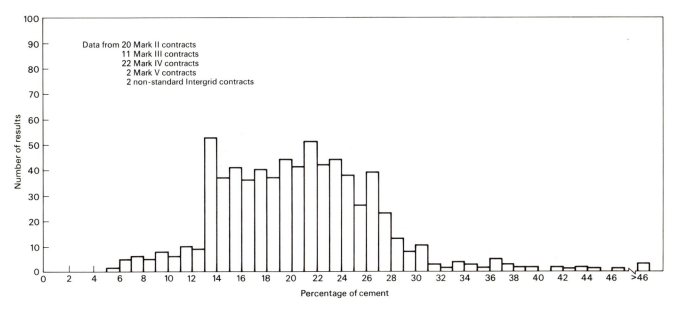

Figure 23 Cement content of samples from precast prestressed beams

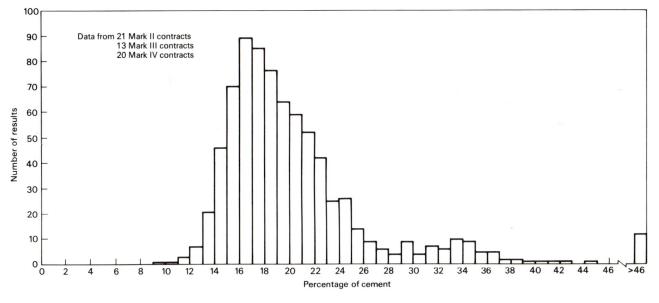

Figure 24 Cement content of samples from pretensioned columns

23

Conclusions

The following conclusions summarise the information drawn from the reports received:

(1) Most components in Intergrid buildings have no visible defects associated with corrosion of tendons or reinforcement. Visible defects (rust staining or cracking) were found on a few beams at 16 sites and on about a quarter of the columns at two sites and on a few columns at 17 sites.

(2) The components in more than two-thirds of Intergrid buildings for which reports were received have low chloride contents. Out of the total of 109 sites, two or more samples from beams in 25 contracts were found to contain at least medium chloride content. For columns, 13 contracts yielded two or more samples with at least medium chloride content. Generally these components were manufactured before 1964.

(3) It is considered that the reported results from beams in nine contracts and from columns in five contracts gave a positive indication that calcium chloride was used in the manufacture of some components. Four manufacturers are believed to have produced some of these components but the manufacturers of the remainder could not be identified. Components at other sites made by the same identified manufacturers had low chloride contents.

(4) Mortar samples taken from Mark II Intergrid beams had low chloride contents. There was no evidence of migration of chlorides into the mortar from the precast concrete.

(5) The precast concrete appears to be of good quality, cement contents generally being above 14 per cent.

(6) The in situ OPC concrete in the joints between the precast units at one site contained high chloride content and at another medium chloride content.

(7) Water penetration causing wet conditions around some beams was reported at five sites.

(8) The relationship between visible defects, tendon corrosion, chloride content and age could not be examined using the limited information in the reports. These relationships are discussed, however, in Section 11 using this information together with that obtained from other parts of the BRE investigation.

6 Investigations of pretensioned Intergrid components

Rust staining, cracking or spalling of the concrete cover was initially brought to the attention of the Building Research Establishment in pretensioned columns of one Mark II Intergrid building in October 1976. Inspection of columns in this structure and similar buildings of like age was made. The structures examined were buildings A to G described below.

Building A was constructed in 1956/57 to the Mark II Intergrid design, partly of single-storey construction but with a two-storey wing and an assembly hall which was of two-storey height. In this building the prestressed concrete columns had shown vertical and horizontal cracking over the two years prior to the inspection. These cracks were associated with corrosion more of the secondary reinforcement located at the ends of the columns than the tendons. Before selecting samples of concrete for analysis, a visual assessment was made of the condition of each column. Of the 133 external columns, some 7 corner columns and 26 side columns were found to be cracked due to corrosion of the tendons and/or secondary reinforcement. It should be noted therefore that cracking showed on about a quarter of the externally exposed columns. In an early visual appraisal of condition, the columns were classified as grey or sandy in appearance, in the belief that concrete quality might be assessed by surface colour. Subsequent examination proved that this was not so.

Following the visual examination, the tendons were exposed in five of the storey-height columns at the top, middle and base. Concrete removed in the process was subsequently analysed for cement and chloride content. Small lengths of tendons were exposed on 10 other columns to assess its condition relative to the surface appearance of the concrete. The depth of carbonation of the concrete was determined at the same time by spraying the freshly exposed concrete surfaces with a solution of phenolphthalein. Concrete samples from uncracked columns were taken by drilling at the top, middle and base sections of storey height columns and from four positions on the taller two-storey height columns. Concrete samples from the internal environment were also taken by drilling the internal face of three of the taller columns.

In all, a total of 15 different columns in building A were sampled by removing sufficient concrete to expose the steel in 32 areas. The extent of corrosion of the steel ranged from substantially nil with only traces of corrosion product on the surface through surface corrosion with pitting, to severe where an estimated 20% or more of the cross-sectional area of the tendon had been lost (Plates 1, 2 and 3). Cracking of the concrete cover had not occurred where slight surface

corrosion was present but became apparent with surface corrosion and pitting. Approximately 60% of the exposed surface areas of the tendons was either covered with a slight rust layer or was uncorroded, 25% had surface corrosion and pitting and the remainder showed severe corrosion with extensive loss of metal. In one case, about 10 mm of the tendon had been destroyed completely.

In general, the greater the cracking of the concrete, the greater was the degree of corrosion on the steel. Cracking was mainly apparent on the external face of the column but at two locations, severe corrosion was accompanied by cracking in the side and re-entrant corner of the column.

Measurement of the depth of carbonation of the concrete gave values from 2 to 15 mm from the surface, the deeper levels (above 12 mm) usually occurring at a corner. At cracks, the carbonation was complete so that at many locations where severe corrosion of the reinforcement had occurred, the surrounding concrete was carbonated. In other locations the steel was found to be surrounded by an alkaline environment even though corrosion had taken place on the tendons. (Plate 4).

Chemical analysis of the samples of concrete indicated cement contents varying from 11.2% to 36.2% with an average of 17.3%, the standard deviation being 3.5%. In any one column the maximum variation found in cement content was 1:2. Generally the cement distribution was reasonably uniform, variation in samples from individual columns usually being less than 1:1.2.

The chloride content of all concrete samples was determined and found to fall between the limits of 0.32% to 6.65% chloride ion by the weight of cement. The average value was 1.60% with a standard deviation of 0.9%. Samples taken from the inside of external columns gave similar chloride concentrations to those samples removed from the external faces. The maximum range of chloride content found in any one column was from 0.32% to 6.65% chloride ion by weight of cement (ie a range of 1:22) but the average range of chloride content in individual components was 1:2.1. The very high variability of chloride content in one column increased the average range. The range was only 1:1.4 or less in many columns, indicating that in general the chloride distribution was reasonably uniform within single components.

In external columns, corrosion of the reinforcement was associated with high levels of chloride content of the concrete. Corrosion was not found necessarily to be associated with the level of chloride content. For example, severe corrosion of reinforcement occurred in three columns with chloride contents of 1.4–3.1%, 0.6–2.2% and 0.5–1.1% chloride ion by weight of the cement respectively, whereas only slight surface corrosion was observed on columns having chloride contents of 0.5–1.1% and 0.7–1.4% similarly exposed (Plate 5).

Internal columns were also examined where accessible. On the limited sample available for inspection, no rust staining or cracking was visible. The inside face of several external columns showed surface crazing, but no cracking which could be associated with corrosion of the reinforcement was observed, even in those columns which had cracking on external faces.

Building B was of similar construction (Mark II Intergrid) and age to building A except that one wing was of three-storey height. Vertical and in some cases horizontal cracking of about a quarter of the columns at their head or base had been observed. Visual inspection revealed that the cracks were deeper than at building A and that there was a greater amount of horizontal cracking. The visual appearance of the concrete was very similar to that at building A. In several columns, cracks were observed which on removing the concrete cover, were found to be the result of deep crazing rather than corrosion of the reinforcement.

Following visual examination, seven cracked columns were selected for further study in order that the condition of the steel could be observed in columns showing defects. Since it was probable that wide cracking of the concrete and corrosion were related, finely cracked columns were selected. Examination of the steel in these seven columns showed that in all but one column the steel was severely corroded with some sections having a thick rust scale and others showing localised pitting corrosion. A tendon in relatively sound condition contained some dark coloured surface markings indicative of the onset of corrosion. Part of the concrete adjacent to this tendon was also carbonated. Pitting corrosion was also detected in one tendon of another column which was examined during the initial inspection of the building. Here, the concrete cover was extensively cracked and could be removed by hand revealing areas on the steel where severe corrosion and considerable loss of cross section had occurred, areas where surface corrosion and pitting had taken place, and areas where there was slight surface corrosion. Whilst the tendon was severely corroded in places there was no evidence of brittleness other than that associated with the reduction in cross-sectional area.

A 10% random sample of ground-floor columns was selected for determination of cement and chloride content and carbonation depth of the concrete. The amounts of chloride found by chemical analyses of the samples were significant, falling within the range 0–2.4% chloride ion by weight of cement, with an average of 1.5% and a standard deviation of 0.56%. Little point-to-point variability in chloride content in individual columns was indicated in the results. The depth of carbonation of the concrete was determined using a phenolpthalein spray at the time and position of sampling. The depth found was within the range 4 to 20 mm from the surface of the concrete. Differential carbonation was observed between the face, side and re-entrant corner of the concrete. In two of the columns examined, carbonation was observed to the depth of embedment of the prestressing tendons. The cement content of the samples ranged from 13% to 19% with a mean of 15.5%, the variation being low within any one column.

Internal columns in building B were visually inspected and no cracking was observed. This inspection was confined to those columns which were readily accessible; in general the concrete surface was painted.

Building C was of Mark II Intergrid construction, built in 1953/54. External columns were of uniform appearance with little evidence of surface crazing. Unlike buildings A and B, no vertical or horizontal cracking at the column heads or bases was apparent. A random 10% sample of ground-floor columns was selected and drilled samples of concrete at two heights in the columns were taken for analysis. The depth of carbonation on the fractured surface between the drilling holes was determined. The maximum depth of carbonation recorded was 2 mm from the exposed face of the concrete although for the majority of the columns sampled, carbonation was less than 1 mm. Concrete samples from 28 columns gave cement contents between 13% and 22% with a mean of 18% cement. Some variation in cement content along individual columns was observed, the worst case giving a variation of 1:1.46. Excluding this column, the variation in other samples did not exceed 1:1.22. The chloride content of the concrete was low, only nine samples, from seven columns, giving a value of over 0.06% chloride ion by weight of the cement. In the nine samples analysed by BRE, the chloride content was between 0.06% and 0.17% chloride ion by weight of cement. Neither the steel tendons nor the reinforcement was exposed at any of the columns in this building. No cracking was observed on visible internal columns.

Building D comprised Mark II and Mark III Intergrid construction with blocks of 1, 2, 3 and 4-storey height. Visual inspection of the external columns revealed none of the vertical cracking observed in building A. There was, however, a pattern of fine horizontal cracking at some column heads. Samples of concrete taken from randomly selected columns showed a variation in chloride content of 0% to 0.3% chloride ion by weight of cement with a mean of 0.06%. Measured carbonation depths were less than 1 mm. In view of the absence of vertical cracking, the sound condition of the columns and the low concentration of chloride ion, no tendons or reinforcement were exposed in the external columns of the building.

Building E was also comprised of Mark II and Mark III Intergrid structures, in this case of single and two-storey construction. Examination of the external columns revealed serious cracking in five columns. Concrete samples, removed from these columns, gave chloride contents ranging from 0% to 5.4% chloride ion by weight of cement with an average value of 2.6%. The concrete was carbonated to depths of 2 mm to 18 mm and had a high porosity. In two of the most severely cracked columns, the tendons were exposed and observed to be severely corroded. A short length of one of these tendons was removed and showed no evidence of brittleness. Tendons were exposed on the uncracked internal faces of columns which had cracked on their externally-exposed surfaces and only surface corrosion was found.

In building F, a multi-storey structure with components of Mark II, Mark III, Mark IV and Mark V Intergrid design, concrete samples were removed from Mark II and Mark IV Intergrid columns. Analyses of the samples from the Mark II columns gave chloride contents of up to 0.3% chloride ion by weight of cement with an average of 0.04%. Depths of carbonation were found to be less than 2 mm. The Mark IV columns showed chloride contents of 0.02% chloride ion by weight of cement.

Building G was of Mark II Intergrid construction built in 1956. Inspection of the external columns revealed that horizontal and vertical cracking had occurred on three columns in the four-storey structure and that some corner columns showed low cover to the secondary reinforcement cages, which had resulted in corrosion sufficient to spall the concrete cover. Near to the top of a few two-storey height columns in one wing of the building there were very fine horizontal cracks which were not thought to be associated with corrosion of embedded metal. Chemical analyses showed that the chloride content of the samples removed from the external columns was up to 1.34% chloride ion by weight of cement and the average cement content was 16.4%. No tendons were exposed in this structure.

Conclusions

From these examinations of pretensioned concrete columns the following conclusions were drawn:

(1) Severe corrosion of parts of the tendons on the external faces of the externally-exposed columns had occurred after about 20 years in service in a substantial proportion of columns where the average chloride content was high, ie above 1.0% chloride ion by weight of cement. The concrete cover was usually carbonated to some extent but severe corrosion was observed in uncarbonated high chloride locations so that carbonation of the concrete is not a prerequisite to corrosion in such areas.

(2) The incidence of corrosion suggested that it could be linked to the quantity of chloride. While this was established qualitatively, the influence of other factors, particularly exposure to moisture and susceptibility to carbonation indicate that it is not possible to quantify precisely a time scale in relation to chloride content associated with corrosion or its relation to easily-measured parameters of the concrete.

(3) A few Intergrid buildings examined contain a level of chloride which can only be attributed to the addition of a chloride-bearing admixture during manufacture. Other Intergrid columns contain a very low quantity of chloride such as could have been introduced in the mix water and cement or by the use of aggregate having a relatively high natural chloride content.

(4) The proportion of columns containing relatively high chloride contents varied with the building contract. Whilst some structures may have chloride added to all columns, the results show that in others only some columns were supplied with high chloride contents.

(5) Exceptionally the distribution of chloride in a given column may be uniform or may vary by as much as 22:1 from one location to another, but usually the variation is about 2:1. Typically the maximum chloride content found in single samples taken from a group of columns was at least twice the mean.

(6) Corrosion of the secondary reinforcement had occurred where the depth of cover was low in a small number of columns where it had been misplaced in manufacture or where the concrete was permeable so that the protective alkalinity of the concrete was reduced by carbonation and/or where the concrete contained a high average chloride content. Permeability of the concrete, as observed by measurement of the depth of carbonation, was often low but on some columns, carbonation had extended to the depth of the embedded steel in 20 years.

(7) Chemical analysis of the concrete samples taken from the concrete indicated that the concrete used contained an extreme range of 11% to 36% cement. Generally the cement distribution was within the range 16% to 20.8%. In general the concrete appeared to be of good quality.

(8) None of the internal columns examined showed signs of corrosion of embedded steel but it was possible only to expose small areas of tendon or reinforcement to verify this observation. The chloride content was similar to that of columns of similar age which had been exposed to an external environment and had cracked due to corrosion of the tendons.

(9) Severe corrosion, resulting from the formation of small but deep pits in the prestressing tendons, was observed at only two sites. In prestressed concrete

columns, externally exposed, it would appear from these examinations that the conditions necessary for such corrosion rarely occur.

(10) In pretensioned columns, externally exposed, the investigations have shown that corrosion of the secondary reinforcement or of the stressed tendon will most probably result in visible signs such as rust staining or cracking of the concrete cover before the components became so weakened as to physically distort or to fail to support the structure above. Columns showing such visible defects are indicative that some corrosion of the embedded steel has occurred and should be thoroughly investigated to determine the cause and consequently what remedial action may be necessary.

(11) There was no evidence of stress corrosion cracking of the tendons in any of the steel examined.

7 Investigations of post-tensioned Intergrid components

Externally stressed post-tensioned beams – Mark II

Limited inspections were carried out by the Establishment of externally-stressed post-tensioned Mark II Intergrid beams in buildings A, B, C, D, F and J. A more extensive inspection of similar beams was possible in building E.

The beams in building A were constructed in 1956/57 to Mark II Intergrid specification and consisted of concrete lattice beams with post-tensioned tendons (diameter 0.276 in) running along the top of the lower flanges. Primary and secondary beams were examined. In the two-storey height structure of the building, five of the primary beams were found to have rust staining on the precast concrete associated with corrosion of the secondary reinforcement arising from a low depth of cover. Close examination of the mortar haunching surrounding the tendons showed no evidence of tendon disruption or of rust staining at the tendon anchor/beam interface. The mortar covering was coated with bitumen paint.

Samples of the precast concrete were removed for analysis. The analyses indicated that the chloride content was equivalent to 0.06% to 0.6% chloride ion by weight of cement with a mean of 0.4%. Small sections of the mortar surrounding the tendons were removed and analysed giving a chloride content of 0.01% to 0.06% chloride ion by weight of cement with a mean of 0.03%. Where exposed the tendons showed slight surface corrosion which may have been present at the time of construction.

Similar beams were examined in building B. Here the protective mortar surrounding the tendons was removed over short lengths up to 100 mm to reveal that the majority of the exposed steel was in very good condition with only small patches of slight surface corrosion. At places, the depth of cover to the tendon was very low and here some surface corrosion and pitting was observed. Surface corrosion was also observed at the steel/steel contact interfaces of groups of tendons which were surrounded by poorly compacted mortar. Chemical analyses of samples of the mortar indicated only traces of chloride, and the depth of carbonation of the mortar was generally less than 3 mm.

In building C the 23-year-old concrete beams consisted of two U-section precast segments joined together to form a square-sectioned unit and then post-tensioned through the central hollow zone. In three of these beams, areas of the mortar cover to the tendons were removed and the steel examined. At each location, the steel had surface corrosion but no pitting or substantial reduction in diameter was observed. Only traces of chloride were found in the mortar surrounding the tendons and this mortar contained between 26% and 29% cement. The mortar was however carbonated to depths of from 7 mm to 12 mm from the top surface (which was not protected by a layer of bitumen paint) but the tendons were still in an alkaline environment. Standard Mark II beams in building C were also examined and the mortar surrounding the tendons found to contain 0.06% to 0.2% chloride ion by weight of cement.

Building D contained Mark II Intergrid beams. There was some evidence of surface corrosion of the tendons. The beam concrete was found to contain 0.45% to 0.51% chloride ion by weight of cement with a mean of 0.47%. Traces of chloride were found to be present in the mortar surrounding the tendons.

Building E was about 19 years old and consisted of Mark II and Mark III Intergrid structures. The Mark II beams were externally post-tensioned, the tendons covered with a cement mortar which had been painted over with bitumen. Chloride ion content of the precast concrete was found ranging from 0% to 0.69% and of the mortar from 0% to 0.01% by weight of the cement. Examination of tendons after removal of mortar showed considerable surface corrosion over some of the tendon surfaces in internal locations where the ambient humidity was high, ie in kitchen and shower areas. This was particularly noticeable at the steel/steel contact surfaces where the tendons were in groups (Plate 6) and also where the mortar covering had been poorly compacted. Similar corrosion was found at the ends of beams where there was no mortar cover to part of the inclined tendons and only bitumen paint had been applied. General surface corrosion, giving an adherent thin rust layer, and flakes of rust, was observed on some areas of the tendons. Rust had formed where the geometry of the metal/concrete interface had prevented complete contact of the mortar around the tendon. Where good contact with the mortar had been established, the steel was effectively free from corrosion but where poor contact obtained the steel was corroded. It would appear that in humid environments moist air had penetrated to the voids around the tendons and condensed there to provide the wet conditions necessary for continued corrosion. Similar corrosion was found to exist in the intersections of primary and secondary beams (Plate 7) and at locations where steel/steel contact was present as, for example, where the post-tensioned tendons change direction in the beam around steel mandrels positioned near their ends (Plate 8).

There was little carbonation of the mortar below the bitumen coating but it had occurred in the mortar adjacent to mortar/concrete and mortar/tendon interfaces at some locations particularly where the mortar had been poorly compacted.

Building F contained Mark II, Mark III and Mark V Intergrid beams. Chemical analysis of concrete samples from the 22-year old Mark II beams gave chloride values from 0.10% to 1.15% chloride ion by weight of the cement. There were no visible signs on the concrete of corrosion of the secondary reinforcement. The mortar surrounding the tendons was found to have chloride contents ranging from 0.11% to 0.17% chloride ion by weight of cement, with a mean value of 0.15%. No corrosion of tendons was reported.

The beams in building J which was built in 1955 were a less common variety of the Mark II Intergrid system in that the tendons ran in channels in the top of the lower flange rather than above the flush surface. In the secondary beams the tendons ran in grooves in the sides of the lower concrete flanges. Inspection of the beams in one part of the structure revealed that in one side-grooved unit the tendon was insufficiently covered by the mortar and showed surface corrosion. Slight rust staining of the concrete at the junctions of primary and secondary beams was observed. In this construction, the tendons of the secondary beams were ducted through the bottom flanges of primary beams: the ducts were not grouted and at some intersections rust staining was evident. Chloride contents of the precast concrete were found ranging from 0% to 0.79% chloride ion by weight of the cement.

Conclusions on externally-stressed post-tensioned beams

The evidence from inspection of tendons in Mark II Intergrid beams up to 23 years old indicated that where corrosion was found it was limited to surface attack except in damp locations. The inspections revealed that at these locations more serious corrosion had developed and that there are some locations in the construction where the tendons are more susceptible to corrosion. Other general conclusions which were drawn from this part of the investigation are:

(1) Most tendons were found to be in good condition but considerable surface corrosion of tendons was observed in some beams. Where present, corrosion on the tendons was in the form of surface rusting in the majority of locations. Rust scale causing a visible loss of cross section of the steel had formed at locations where there was poor compaction of the mortar cover. No severe pitting corrosion of the tendons was observed.

(2) In internal situations such as in kitchens or shower areas where the ambient humidity may be high, the degree of corrosion was greater due to the greater moisture content of the surrounding mortar caused by condensation.

(3) There are locations in the construction where the tendons are more susceptible to corrosion. These locations include the junction between primary and secondary beams, changes in direction of the tendons (as around steel mandrels near the ends of beams) and areas where several tendons are grouped together. At all these locations the embedment of the tendons in the surrounding

mortar has not always provided an adequate protection against corrosion.

(4) Lack of cover of tendons in the mortar at some locations has resulted in considerable surface rusting. The bitumen paint coating alone has been insufficient to prevent this corrosion.

(5) In some buildings the mortar is permeable and poorly compacted around the tendons and the depth of cover is low. Corrosion of tendons has occurred under these conditions even though the chloride content of the mortar is low. There is an appreciable depth of carbonation of the mortar at some locations which are not protected by a bitumen coating, even though the cement content is high. Carbonation of the mortar has occurred adjacent to mortar/concrete and mortar/tendon interfaces at some locations.

(6) There was no evidence of significant migration of chloride ions from the precast concrete into the mortar. The chloride content of the mortar was less than 0.2% chloride ion by weight of the cement.

(7) Tendon corrosion in these internal beams was very much less advanced than in some exposed pretensioned columns. This has probably arisen partly because of the lower chloride content of the embedding mortar in beams and partly because of the much drier conditions indoors. Sufficient humidity could be present indoors to allow considerable corrosion of the tendons to occur in some locations.

Internally stressed post-tensioned beams

During the investigations by the Establishment evidence was obtained from three Intergrid sites and a monitor beam structure of the condition of post-tensioned beams and their internally-stressed tendons. The sites were designated H, R, W and T.

The building at site H was constructed in 1959 using prototype Mark III post-tensioned beams comprising three precast elements and spanning forty feet.

The condition of the beams as assessed by visual inspection was good with only slight evidence of corrosion of a few stirrups which had very low cover locally and of some pipe ducts cast into the webs to support the false ceilings. However visual inspection revealed that a group of three beams had deflections which could not be explained by analysis or load considerations. It was therefore decided to investigate the condition of the tendons and to sample the concrete for chemical analysis. Cores 50 mm in diameter were cut from the sides of the beams at the level of the tendons at mid-span and in the in-situ concrete forming the joints between the precast beam elements.

The ducts at mid-span were found to be slightly corroded but at the joints some had suffered surface attack and one had been perforated whilst others were bright. Removal of the steel duct at the base of the cored holes showed the tendons to be apparently dry but surface corroded at all locations. Generally the ducts appeared to be completely filled with grout except at mid-span in two beams which were partially filled (Plate 9) and one duct which had no grout at either mid-span or at one of the insitu joints.

The chloride content of the concrete was determined by analyses of the cores. Up to 1.6% chloride ion by weight of cement was found in one precast component and the results were in the range 1.1% to 1.6% chloride ion by weight of cement for the in-situ joint concrete. Chloride content of the grout was up to 0.06% chloride ion by weight of cement. These results suggested that calcium chloride was added to one of the precast beam sections and to the in-situ concrete forming the joints between the precast beam elements.

The building at site R was constructed in 1959 using Mark III post-tensioned beams for the floor and roof structures. The primary beams were believed to be supplied by two manufacturers and chloride contents in the precast concrete were less than 0.3% chloride ion by weight of cement. The condition of the beams, which are in an internal environment, appeared good on visual inspection and inspection of the condition of the duct and tendons revealed no evidence of active corrosion of the ducts or the tendons. The ducts appeared to be completely filled with grout and analyses of grout samples indicated traces of chloride only. Visual inspection of the secondary beams indicated slight corrosion of secondary reinforcement at points of no cover. These secondary beams were found to have only traces of chloride present in the concrete.

The building at site W, constructed in 1961/62, was a non standard Intergrid structure consisting of 12 post-tensioned prestressed concrete roof beams 60 ft long placed 25 ft apart, spanning between reinforced concrete columns and supporting precast reinforced concrete purlins which in turn supported a corrugated metal decking and weather-proofing system. Collapse of a prestressed roof beam occurred without warning in 1974. The subsequent investigation revealed that the collapse had been caused by failure of the internal post-tensioned tendons (3 no. ducts each containing 12 no. 0.276 in diameter wire) following severe corrosion associated with the presence of chlorides and moisture in the beam which comprised three precast units.

The chloride content of the three precast units from the beam that failed were:

	Number of samples	Range of chloride content (% chloride ion by weight of cement)
End unit A	3	0.38 to 0.75
Mid unit B	17	0.43 to 0.75
End unit C	25	0.45 to 2.62

The tendons failed at the junction of the end unit C and middle unit B. In the immediate vicinity of this joint the average chloride contents were 1.24% chloride ion by weight of cement for end unit C and 0.33% for the middle unit B. The average chloride contents in twelve grout samples taken from the modules adjacent to the joint were 0.82% for end unit C and 0.10% for the middle unit B. The highest recorded chloride content in the grout adjacent to the joint between units A and B was 0.04% chloride ion by weight of cement. It was found that the ducts had not been completely filled with grout and they were wet inside (Plate 10). In the vicinity of the failure at the joint between units C and B the mild steel duct had been corroded through in many places (Plate 11) and the connector in the duct liner at the beam joint was not designed to be watertight. There was therefore no difficulty in chloride ions from the precast concrete reaching the tendons.

The precast unit which had the highest chloride contents (unit C) had some cracking with brown rust staining at a few locations which was associated with corrosion of the secondary reinforcement (Plate 12). There were also areas of repair where the concrete had been 'made good' probably at the time of manufacture. The minimum cement content of the concrete in the beam was 17% and it was found that the depth of carbonation was up to 18 mm.

The building at site T was a monitor structure constructed in 1964 using five monitor beams similar to that shown in Figure 15. The building was clad mainly in thin gauge metal or translucent sheeting and by brick infill between columns up to a height of about 1.5 m.

On visual inspection the beams appeared to be in good condition except for rust stains on the in-situ concrete surfaces at the joints between the precast units in top booms. In some cases the staining appeared to come from the interfaces between the precast and in situ concrete. Unfortunately it was not possible at the time to remove concrete locally at the affected joints to examine the condition of the embedded steel.

The chloride content of the precast concrete was found to be in the range 0.5% to 0.9% chloride ion by weight of the cement and that of the in-situ joint concrete was up to 0.32% chloride ion by weight of the cement. These results suggested that calcium chloride was added during manufacture of the precast concrete.

The stability of the structure against lateral forces appeared to be ensured by the precast concrete purlins which were bolted to the monitor beams by four bolts and possibly by two longitudinal edge beams at the eaves of the monitor beams and by fixity at the base of the columns. Visual inspection suggested that the structure might be sensitive to extensive collapse should failure of the post-tensioned tendons occur in one beam.

Conclusions on internally-stressed post-tensioned beams

The following conclusions were drawn from the investigations of internally-stressed post-tensioned beams:

(1) Severe corrosion of tendons was apparent in one beam following failure (Site W). The limited investigation of the condition of tendons in other beams revealed surface corrosion only. It was not possible to determine whether this surface attack was progressing.

(2) Corrosion of tendons may occur locally and lead to sudden fracture before a major proportion of tendon length is affected.

(3) The rate at which deterioration of tendons can occur as a result of corrosion cannot be estimated accurately. This topic is discussed in Section 11.

(4) Corrosion of secondary reinforcement causing cracking and rust staining of the precast concrete may occur giving a visible indication that the tendons may be corroding. The evidence was insufficient to confirm that such visible signs will always develop at the same time or prior to the occurrence of severe local tendon corrosion and sudden tendon fracture.

(5) Steel ducts cannot be assumed to be completely filled with grout or to prevent the migration of chloride ions from the concrete to the tendons. The known environment of the component and the local environment in the vicinity of the tendon are not necessarily similar.

(6) High or medium chloride content may exist in the precast concrete units or in the in-situ concrete at joints in Intergrid beams. In these circumstances corrosion of tendons may be more likely to occur in the vicinity of the joints and may be indicated by rust staining on the concrete surface.

(7) Carbonation had occurred in one case to a depth of 18 mm in 12 years.

(8) A few Intergrid structures with internal post-tensioned tendons may be more sensitive than others to extensive collapse in the event of failure of tendons in one beam.

8 Investigations of components from other concrete structures

One aim of the BRE investigation was to try to examine possible relationships between the condition of tendons and the age of components in Intergrid buildings in terms of the main factors affecting the ability of the concrete cover to protect the embedded steel from corrosion. Such relationships would be valuable, if established, in assessments of the present and future condition of these buildings. Clearly no precise forecast can be made of the likely future condition of Intergrid buildings during their intended life since the information now obtained is from one examination in time only and experience does not extend beyond 23 years. Information on performance in service of components in other concrete structures was sought therefore to compare with that on Intergrid components and to provide a wider basis for commenting on future possible performance. Two types of component were examined:

1 Pretensioned concrete, and
2 Precast reinforced concrete.

The majority of these components were examined as a result of deterioration in service and were therefore not representative of components in buildings in general.

1 Pretensioned concrete components

With the assistance of owners two batches of pretensioned components which had been in service for a considerable time were obtained from two sources. The components had been subjected to external exposure, one batch having been used as masts supporting overhead cables and the other as railway sleepers.

Pretensioned masts.

Masts which had been manufactured in 1950/51 were delivered to the Building Research Station from an outside store where they had been since removal from service in 1972. The reason for their removal from service was reported to be cracking between the flanges and the webs due to poor detailing. They were tapered pretensioned 'I' sections reinforced with nominal 5 mm diameter indented high tensile prestressing tendons and 11 mm square twisted steel reinforcing bars (Figure 25). Two masts about 8 m long were examined in detail by visual inspection initially and during removal of the concrete cover, by chemical analyses of the concrete and by tests on the tendons.

The cover at the flange face to the prestressing tendons in the masts was found to be 22 mm to 33 mm and the cover to the square twisted bars at the web/flange intersection was 8 mm to 16 mm. Longitudinal cracking of the concrete was present at the junction between the flanges and webs and also in the first mast along the centre of one flange. Whilst the former was probably initiated by structural stress due to poor detailing the latter was most probably caused by the expansion products of corrosion. Throughout the two masts the tendons had slight surface rusting which was not associated with any visible concrete cracking. However

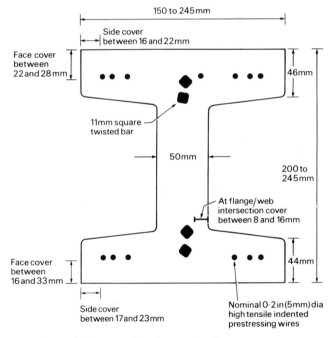

Figure 25 Typical cross-section of pretensioned mast

extensive surface corrosion and pitting of the tendons had occurred at locations in the flanges of the first mast, increasing the apparent diameter of the 5.1 mm tendons to about 5.5 mm associated with longitudinal hair cracks (0.05 mm wide) at the concrete surface. Where corrosion was severe, ie cross sectional area reduced by 20 % or more, a crack about 2 mm wide ran adjacent to and for the same length as the corroded part of the tendon. The tendons adjacent to those which were severely attacked showed signs of local deterioration themselves. This may have been due to cracking induced at these locations lowering the protection to the adjacent tendons. In the second mast corrosion was restricted to slight surface rusting of tendons with some patches of surface corrosion and pitting; no substantial reductions in cross-sectional area were found.

Chemical analyses of samples of the concrete indicated chloride contents varying in the first mast from 0.4% to 0.7% and in the second mast from 0.2% to 0.4% chloride ion by weight of cement with cement contents in the range 20.7% to 26.3%. The range of chloride results was similar in both flanges of the first mast and although the average chloride content was higher in the flange which contained the most serious corrosion, ie 0.6% compared with 0.4% chloride ion by weight of cement, it cannot be said that this difference accounted for the difference in corrosion present. Likewise it cannot be said with confidence that the difference in corrosion between the two masts is accounted for by the difference in chloride content since some enhancement of corrosion by carbonation along cracks may have occurred.

The depth of carbonation of the concrete from the outer exposed surfaces was small in both masts, ie less than 1 mm, as measured by the phenolphthalein test. Carbonation had occurred however along the sides of cracks, in some cases extending to the steel, and may have played some part in subsequent corrosion. Samples of the concrete were found to have a low porosity.

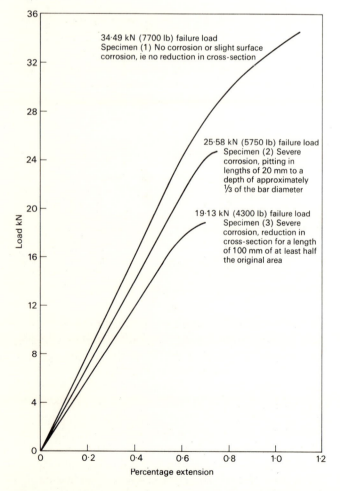

Figure 26 Load/extension curves for specimens of corroded high tensile prestressing tendon (indented)

34

The remaining prestress in the tendons was found to be lower (0.40 fy to 0.46 fy) than would normally be expected (normal design figure is 0.52 fy). This indicates that either the tendons were not fully stressed in the first instance or the losses which occurred in practice were greater than those assumed in design – a factor which has been noted previously[23]. These greater losses in practice may be a general phenomenon not associated with corroded tendons.

Load/strain curves were obtained by tests on tendon samples selected to represent different degrees of corrosion. Typical curves are shown in Figure 26 which indicate that the load carrying capacity reduced with the degree of corrosion and, as might be expected, local corrosion of the tendons changed their extension characteristics under load. Whether failure of a pretensioned component is brittle or ductile will depend however, on the relative location of areas of corrosion in the individual tendons and the extent to which bond with the concrete is retained.

The conclusions from the study of the masts were:

(1) Severe corrosion of parts of tendons in a completely exposed pretensioned component accompanied by cracking of the concrete occurred in 26 years when the concrete contained 0.4% to 0.7% chloride ion by weight of cement and a high cement content (greater than 20%) and there was a very low depth of carbonation from the concrete surface. In a similar component containing chloride content in the range 0.2% to 0.4% chloride ion by weight of cement surface corrosion was present after similar exposure.

(2) Corrosion of tendons had progressed locally leading to the most severe corrosion being concentrated in particular locations.

(3) Variation in the concrete cover in the range of 25 mm to 35 mm did not appear to be a major factor in the distribution of corrosion in the components.

Railway Sleepers.

Five pretensioned concrete railway sleepers manufactured in 1950 using a limestone aggregate and which had been exposed to the weather in the track were examined. The concrete was found to be very hard and uncracked and carbonation had not penetrated more than 1 mm from the surface. Chloride contents of the concrete were less than 0.16% chloride ion by weight of cement and the cement content was 17%. The tendons were exposed by breaking away the surrounding concrete. They were dull grey in appearance and showed no signs of corrosion.

The examination of the railway sleepers showed that external exposure of good quality pretensioned concrete components with chloride ion content less than 0.2% by weight of cement did not lead to corrosion over a period of 27 years.

2 Precast reinforced concrete components

Precast components used as cladding panels at sites K, L and M, as roof planks at site P and as roof purlins at site Q were examined.

Site K Cladding Panels

These panels were 7 ft × 3 ft 4 in (2.13 m × 1.01 m) rectangular panels manufactured and erected in 1966 on low-rise buildings. The panels consist of a thin concrete membrane ($\frac{3}{8}$ in) with a thicker section around the perimeter ($2\frac{1}{4}$ in × $2\frac{1}{4}$ in) containing a single $\frac{3}{8}$ in diameter plain steel bar, except along the bottom of each panel where two bars formed the perimeter reinforcement, and where a further bar had been inserted to provide additional reinforcement to the slots in which fixing angle brackets were placed. Depth of cover to the steel ranged from a minimum of 10 mm (along the bottom of the panels and elsewhere in the perimeter where the bar was close to a weather grooving) to a maximum of 30 mm from the panel face. The concrete was made with limestone aggregate and the panels were finished with Derbyshire spar chippings.

Prior to the examination cracking had become apparent around the perimeter of several panels, especially along their bases, and one panel became detached from its fixings and had fallen from the wall. A number of panels of similar type were examined and approximately 15% showed cracking at the perimeter. Three panels were removed from one building, two showed cracking prior to removal, and the third cracked during the removal process; all had seriously corroded reinforcement. Samples of concrete were taken by drilling panels on a number of buildings to provide data on the chloride content. The limestone aggregate precluded an accurate measure of the cement content of the concrete. However, on the assumption that the specified $1:4\frac{1}{2}$ mix had been used the chloride contents ranged from 0.02% to 2.05% chloride ion by weight of the cement with a mean from 42 samples of 0.49%.

Carbonation tests were carried out on samples from the removed panels. All showed significant carbonation usually to a depth in excess of 10 mm and, in the majority of cases to the depth of the reinforcement from the nearest exposed surface. In the remainder of cases carbonation depths had reached very close to the steel.

The following comments are relevant:

(1)   Corrosion of the reinforcing steel led to cracking of the perimeter concrete in less than 10 years.
(2)   Chloride was present in most panels.
(3)   Considerable carbonation had occurred indicating low-quality concrete of high permeability.
(4)   The combined effect of the panel design, extensive carbonation, and the presence of chloride in the concrete had led to corrosion of the reinforcement, but the contribution of each of these factors could not be determined.

Site L: Cladding Panels

These rectangular cladding panels on three single-storey buildings ranged in approximate size from 6 ft to 23 ft × $3\frac{1}{2}$ ft (1.82 m to 7.01 m × 1.07 m). Their design included a reinforced perimeter stiffening rib, and on the larger panels intermediate reinforced stiffening ribs. The centre, thinner, membrane was unreinforced. They were constructed in 1967–68. During the last 3 years horizontal and vertical cracking, spalling and rust-staining associated with corrosion of the reinforcement have become apparent. The deterioration is now extensive with at least two-thirds of the panels affected.

Approximately ten per cent of the panels, ie 20 panels, were chosen at random and drilled to provide samples of concrete for analyses of cement and chloride contents. The cement contents ranged from 13% to 17% and the chloride contents from 0.10% to 4.32% chloride ion by weight of the cement with a mean chloride ion content of 1.96%. Five of the 20 panels were uncracked. The chloride contents of the cracked panels ranged from 0.98% to 4.32% and that of the uncracked panels from 0.10% to 2.14% chloride ion by weight of cement.

In a number of areas adjacent to corroded reinforcement the concrete had spalled from the panels and these were tested for carbonation using phenolphthalein indicator solution. In the main, the fractured surfaces resulting from corrosion spalling were fully carbonated and tests on freshly-fractured surfaces at right angles to the face of the concrete and the line of spalling indicated carbonation up to 20 mm in depth from the exposed front face and some carbonation from the corrosion-fracture faces. These observations indicated that the concrete was of high permeability.

From this examination it was found that:

(1)   Cracking of the concrete to the depth of the reinforcement had occurred in cladding panels resulting from severe corrosion of reinforcing steel.
(2)   Carbonation of the concrete in panels which had spalled as a result of corrosion of the reinforcement was up to 20 mm in depth.
(3)   The concrete in the majority of the panels contained a high chloride content.
(4)   The majority of panels containing chloride in concentrations above 1.0% chloride ion showed cracking.

Site M: Cladding Panels

These exposed aggregate panels, 2 ft 6 in × 5 ft 3 in (0.76 m × 1.60 m) and 2 ft 6 in × 3 ft (0.76 m × 0.91 m), having a uniform thickness of 2 in (50 mm) form the facade of a 10-storey building constructed in about 1955. They are secured to the building by cast-in concrete nibs which form part of the internal walls.

Recent inspection of the cladding panels revealed vertical and horizontal cracking in a number of them. A full survey followed which indicated that about 26% of the panels were cracked. The cracking appeared to be associated with wire mesh reinforcement in the panels. Removal of cracked concrete cover revealed rusting steel, some of which was severely corroded. As a consequence chemical analyses for chloride content and depth of carbonation of the concrete in the panels were made on samples from about 3% of the panels. Analyses of six samples gave cement contents of 14.4%, 15.5%, 17.2%, 17.4%, 18.0% and 19.9%. The average value was 17.1%, the value on which chloride ion concentrations have been calculated. These values ranged from 0.10% to 3.07% chloride ion by weight of cement with a mean value of 1.55%. The lowest chloride ion content in a cracked panel was 0.51%, and the highest chloride ion content in an uncracked panel was 2.72%.

Tests on freshly-fractured surfaces on a number of the concrete samples which had been removed from cracked areas of panels indicated that much of the steel would have been in alkaline concrete were it not for the cracking associated with corrosion of the reinforcement. However the depth of carbonation was almost 10 mm in some cases. The minimum depth of cover was 12 mm in places.

The observations can be summarised:
(1) The corrosion of the steel was severe at some locations and was associated with cracking of the concrete cover.
(2) The chloride content of the panels was high, the average content for all the panels being above the 1.0% chloride ion content recommended in earlier Codes of Practice.
(3) Carbonation, though extensive, had not in general reached the depths of the steel reinforcement.

Site P: Roof Planks

These were hollow planks, approximately 6 ft × 1 ft × 8 in (1.83 m × 0.30 m × 0.20 m) in size, reinforced by plain ⅜ in (9.5 mm) mild steel bar. The planks formed the roof deck of a two-storey structure, and were covered with a mortar screed and an asphalt topping. The building was erected in 1938.

Parts of the roof had suffered persistent leaks throughout its life, and during a recent redecoration, plasterers discovered ceiling cracks which penetrated to the depth of the reinforcement. Removal of the cover revealed corrosion of the reinforcement.

During a preliminary visit to the building two samples of concrete were taken from the same apparently-dry area of roof, one from a location adjacent to surface corroded and one adjacent to severely corroded bars. Chemical analyses indicated 10.5% and 10.15% cement

and 0.01% and 0.62% chloride ion by weight of cement in the two samples respectively. Tests on freshly-fractured surfaces of the concrete indicated carbonation depths of between 15 mm and 30 mm in the first sample and between 10 mm and 20 mm in the second sample. In the former case carbonation had passed beyond the depth of cover and in the latter the bar had remained in an alkaline environment.

Site Q: Roof Purlins

These 20 ft (6.09 m) long precast concrete purlins were approximately 35 years old and normally reinforced with plain mild steel bars. The cross-section was 'T' shaped with one 25 mm diameter bar in the bottom and two 12 mm diameter bars in the top and shear stirrups were provided at 100 mm centres along the length.

The purlins were covered with a pattern of long hair cracks. In almost every case the cracks ran parallel to a reinforcing bar which was corroding underneath; the position of the steel could be plotted by following the crack pattern. The width and extent of cracking was uniform over the whole length of the purlins. The chloride content was high giving results between 1.0% and 1.9% chloride ion by weight of cement. The cement content was found to be between 15% and 19%.

One purlin was broken up with some difficulty and the concrete tested for carbonation and the reinforcing cage examined. Carbonation had taken place to a depth of between 25 mm and 40 mm along the entire length of the purlin. In some locations it had penetrated along the length via holes cast in the web causing carbonation to extend across the whole width of the section. Samples of the concrete were found to have a high porosity compared to that in the pretensioned masts. Considerable surface corrosion of the reinforcing steel extending to a depth of about 0.5 mm below the original bar surfaces had taken place evenly on those parts of the bars which were in the carbonated zone of the concrete. The worst surface rusting was observed on the 25 mm bars, but because of their large diameter, had not significantly reduced their cross-sectional area.

The following conclusions were drawn:
(1) Serious corrosion can occur in components made of concrete with high chloride content after carbonation in internal apparently – dry conditions.
(2) Carbonation can occur to the depth of steel reinforcement in apparently sound concrete in a period of 35 years.
(3) The corrosion was probably due mainly to carbonation which resulted in almost uniform attack of the steel surfaces generally producing long hair-cracks in the concrete parallel to the reinforcement.

Relevant conclusions from the investigations of precast reinforced concrete components

The findings on reinforced concrete components containing chloride have similarities with the observations on some Intergrid buildings in terms of cement and chloride contents and depths of carbonation. At only one of these sites (Site P) was the cement content considerably lower than the minimum found in Intergrid buildings. General conclusions which can be drawn from this series of investigations are:

(1) A relationship between concrete cracking (associated with corrosion of reinforcement) and chloride content was not established. Cracking was not always present in concrete containing high levels of chloride and cracking was observed in some concrete containing medium levels of chloride.

(2) Where the concrete had a high chloride content corrosion of reinforcement sufficient to cause cracking of the surrounding concrete had occurred in 22 years of external exposure but has been apparent at ages within 10 years of construction.

(3) In an external environment corrosion of reinforcing steel can occur where the depth of carbonation is less than the depth of cover to the steel and where the concrete has a high chloride content.

(4) In an apparently-dry internal environment, corrosion of embedded steel sufficient to cause cracking of the concrete may occur in about 35 years due to the carbonation of the concrete and the presence of a high chloride content. The time scale for corrosion in components in an internal environment is longer than for similar components subject to external exposure.

(5) Chloride content, carbonation of the concrete and exposure to moisture have been confirmed as major factors associated with corrosion of reinforcement. Where chloride content is the dominant factor corrosion tends to vary in severity along the reinforcement compared to a more uniform attack in carbonated concrete. Carbonation becomes more important with increasing age. The time scale associated with corrosion cannot be defined precisely in any particular case.

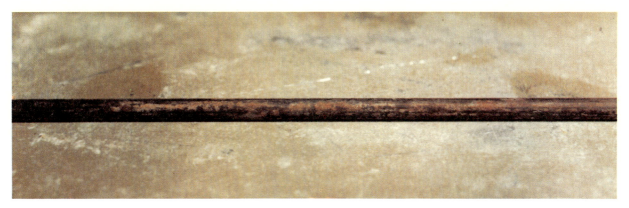

Plate 1 Tendon with slight surface corrosion. No visible loss of area of sound metal at any one cross-section

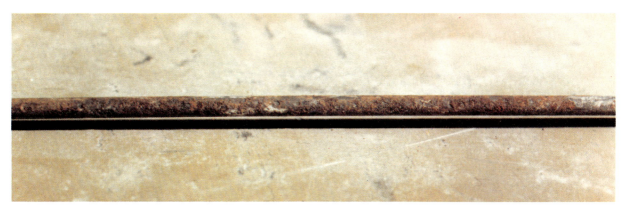

Plate 2 Tendon with surface corrosion and pitting at the onset of visible loss of cross-sectional area of sound metal. Small reduction of tensile strength possible

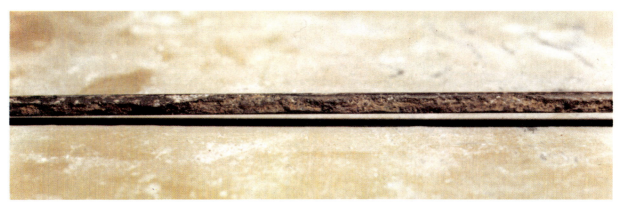

Plate 3 Severely corroded tendon. Estimated 20% or more of area at any one cross-section and corresponding reduction of tensile strength

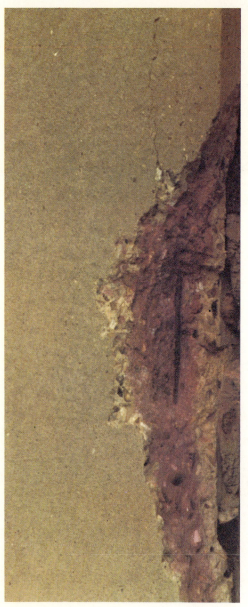
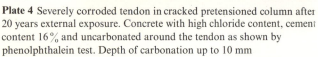
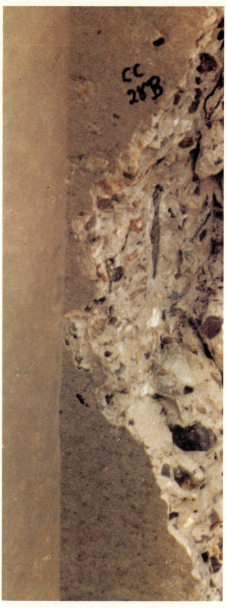

Plate 4 Severely corroded tendon in cracked pretensioned column after 20 years external exposure. Concrete with high chloride content, cement content 16% and uncarbonated around the tendon as shown by phenolphthalein test. Depth of carbonation up to 10 mm

Plate 5 Slight surface corrosion in uncracked pretensioned column after 20 years external exposure. Concrete with high chloride content and cement content 17%

Plate 6 Surface corrosion of external tendons and poor compaction of mortar around tendons revealed after removal of mortar cover in Mark II Intergrid beam. Age 18 years. Mortar partially carbonated with chloride content less than 0.1% ion by weight of cement

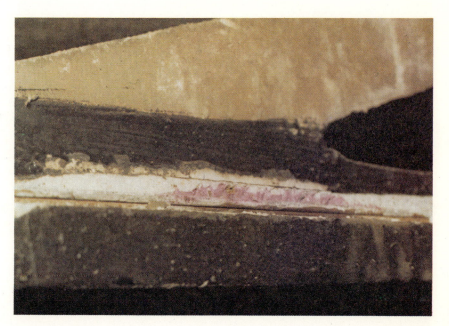

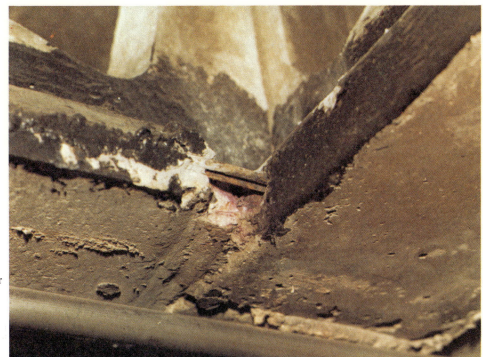

Plate 7 Surface corrosion of external tendons revealed after removal of mortar at intersection of Mark II Intergrid beams. Age 18 years. Mortar poorly compacted and partially carbonated with chloride content less than 0.1 % ion by weight of cement

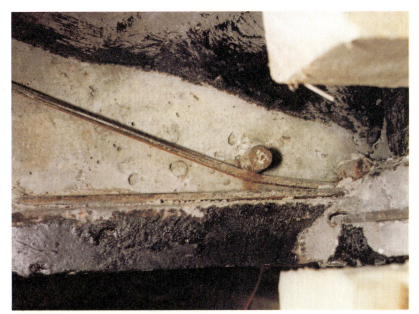

Plate 8 Surface corrosion of external tendons revealed after removal of mortar at end of Mark II Intergrid beam. Age 18 years. Mortar poorly compacted and partially carbonated with chloride content less than 0.1 % chloride ion by weight of cement

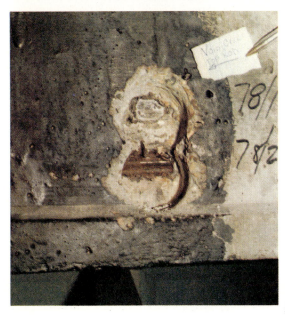

Plate 9 Internal tendons exposed at joint in post-tensioned beam showing surface corrosion of tendons in lower duct and void in upper part of lower duct. Age 18 years

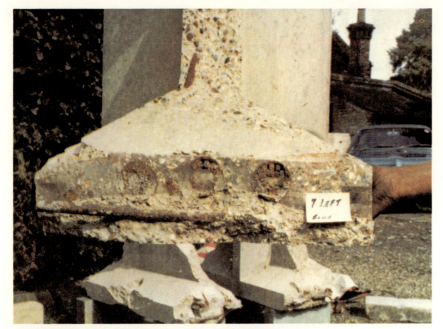

Plate 10 Sawn cross-section of post-tensioned beam after collapse in a non standard Intergrid building showing incomplete grouting of internal tendons. Age 12 years

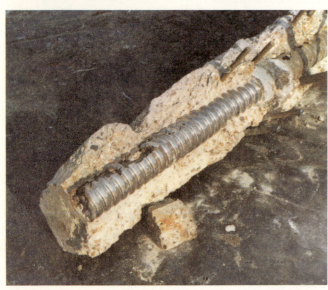

Plate 11 Length of duct and tendons removed from a beam after collapse in a non standard building showing incomplete grouting of duct, penetration of duct wall by corrosion from the inside and the bright external surface of the duct in the foreground compared to the adjacent corroded surface at the other side of the joint in the background. Age 12 years. High chloride content in concrete

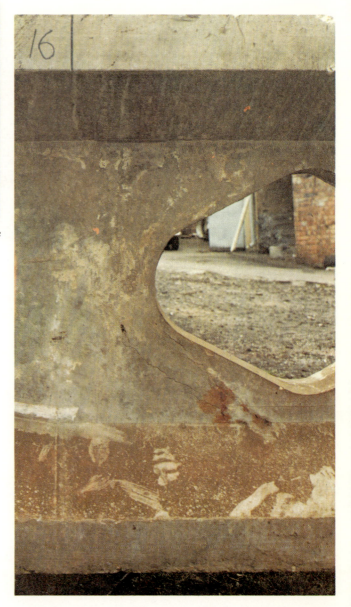

Plate 12 Post-tensioned beam from a non standard building with internal tendons showing rust staining and cracking caused by corrosion of secondary reinforcement. Age 12 years. High chloride content in concrete

9 Inspection techniques

In addition to providing an opportunity of assessing the condition of Intergrid buildings in service as reported in Sections 6 and 7, the work undertaken by the Building Research Establishment at sites in collaboration with owners and their representatives enabled experience of the effectiveness of several inspection techniques for prestressed concrete structures to be obtained. Experience was also obtained from the laboratory and field investigation of other prestressed components and of reinforced components described in Section 8. In addition a study was made of techniques used in other fields to determine their usefulness for inspection of prestressed Intergrid structures. The inspection techniques which were examined may be considered under the following headings:

(1) visual inspection
(2) sampling and testing techniques to determine the quality and condition of concrete, mortar or grout, and
(3) techniques for determining the condition of embedded prestressing tendons.

1 Visual inspection

The present examination of the condition of Intergrid buildings arose as the result of identification of defects during visual inspection. Subsequently, and in common with general structural engineering experience, visual inspection has been found to be a valuable technique for obtaining an early indication of the condition of Intergrid structures and in indicating the most important aspects for further investigation. Apart from enabling defects due to other causes, eg structural movement, mechanical damage or patching of concrete during manufacture, to be found, early indications of the presence of tendon corrosion were obtained in some types of Intergrid component. In one case the identification of untoward deflections of beams indicated the need for further investigation.

Clearly, the nature of the construction must be borne in mind during a visual inspection. Important factors are the sensitivity of the structure to defects and the type of defect which may be associated with the particular construction being examined. For example very fine cracks may be of no significance in reinforced concrete structures, but in prestressed concrete construction they indicate that conditions in the structure have departed substantially from the design and should be investigated. Likewise transverse cracking in beams in reinforced concrete construction may be associated with structural movements or corrosion of transverse reinforcement whereas longitudinal cracks may indicate corrosion of longitudinal steel. Rust stains on concrete surfaces should be examined with care to establish their cause. In prestressed concrete construction they may indicate severe corrosion of tendons or secondary reinforcement, in the immediate vicinity and possibly elsewhere.

For pretensioned Intergrid columns, cracking, rust staining or spalling was seen in cases where, on removal of concrete cover, corrosion of the embedded tendons or secondary reinforcement was found. Removal of concrete cover at locations where no visible defects were seen initially on the concrete surface revealed tendons with no corrosion or only slight surface corrosion.

For Mark II beams with external post-tensioned tendons, rust stains were found at a few locations on precast elements (usually associated with corrosion of secondary reinforcement) and at joints but these stains gave no reliable indication of the condition of the tendons. Visual inspection of mortar in Mark II structures which was usually covered by bitumen paint likewise gave no reliable indication of the condition of the tendons beneath.

For beams with internal post-tensioned tendons, there was no reliable visible sign to indicate tendon corrosion although in the one case where a beam failed due to tendon corrosion subsequent examination of photographic evidence, eg Plate 12, suggested that rust stains on the concrete surface associated with corrosion of the secondary reinforcement would have indicated, if visual inspection for corrosion had been made prior to the failure, that tendon corrosion might have been present. In one building, rust stains were observed at the joints between precast units but it was not possible to examine the condition of the adjacent embedded steel.

2 Sampling and testing techniques to determine the condition and quality of concrete, mortar or grout

Since there may be considerable variation in the quality of the concrete and the chloride content in any one building it was suggested in the annex to the Department's letters (Appendix A) and in Information

Sheet IS 13/77[4] that samples be taken from 10% of beams and columns in each storey with a minimum of three samples being taken where there are less than 30 components in any storey. A similar sampling frequency was suggested for mortar in externally-stressed beams and attention was drawn to the desirability of taking samples from any individual components whose failure might cause major collapse of the building.

This sampling frequency, which was determined from consideration of the manufacturing techniques and the sizes of building involved, was intended to act as a screening process in order to provide a reasonably high probability of identifying batches of components in a building where high chloride contents were present and thus to indicate possible areas for more detailed investigation. BRE experience so far suggests that this level of screening is appropriate. However, high amounts of chloride have been found subsequently in some of the in-situ O.P.C. concrete used in jointing precast elements to form beam components in some Intergrid buildings (see Section 7). It would therefore be prudent to sample this in-situ material also as a part of an assessment of the risk of tendon corrosion in Intergrid buildings.

Drilling the concrete with a masonry bit was found to be the most convenient method of taking concrete samples for subsequent chemical analysis and detailed recommendations for this method and also for chipped samples were made in Information Sheet IS 13/77[4]. Further experience suggested that these recommendations are satisfactory.

Chemical analyses of concrete samples for chloride and cement content in accordance with BS 1881: Part 6 were suggested in the Department's letters. In view of the cost of these analyses and the numbers required for screening of large buildings, investigation of simplified and cheaper methods for use in screening for chloride content was undertaken.

Two simplified techniques for chloride analysis resulted, the 'Quantab' method[3] and the 'Hach' test[4], which required only simple apparatus and were suitable for site use. Table 2 gives a comparison of typical results of tests by the British Standard and simplified methods, and shows a reasonable agreement between results from the three methods. The simplified and approximate procedures used in the 'Quantab' and 'Hach' test methods are therefore capable of providing a satisfactory estimate of the chloride levels in concrete for screening purposes, but where the results are of greater significance, and with doubtful or borderline cases, the more accurate British Standard method for chloride analysis should be employed. Experience reported to date has indicated successful use of the simplified methods both in field and laboratory tests, the results obtained generally showing good agreement with those of occasional check tests by the British Standard method for chloride determination. However, in one report of tests it was observed that the chloride values found on site by the 'Hach' method were about

three times the corresponding chloride contents subsequently determined in the laboratory by the British Standard method. It is possible that this discrepancy was connected with failure to use representative test samples of powdered concrete in the two methods. In another reported instance, erroneous results were obtained by the 'Quantab' method owing to additions of an incorrect quantity of sodium carbonate so that the acid extract was not neutralised before testing. Where there is a danger of such an occurrence the acidity or alkalinity, as appropriate, of the extracts from the concrete sample should be checked by means of an indicator test paper.

When determination of the cement content in hardened Portland cement concrete is required, it appears that the procedure based on chemical analysis of the concrete sample for calcium oxide generally provides a satisfactory estimate of cement content. In one series of tests, however, unreasonably low values for cement content in the region of 5%, or less, were frequently found by the procedure described in Clause 4.1.1.1 of BS 1881: Part 6, and it is likely that excessive additions of sodium hydroxide solution were sometimes made resulting in precipitation of calcium hydroxide from the solution and causing low results for soluble calcium oxide and hence for cement content. This effect can be avoided by using a pH meter to control the addition of sodium hydroxide solution so as to give a pH value of 3 to 4 before adding the solid sodium succinate. Alternatively, as indicated in reference (3), the method described in Clause 6.2 of BS 4550: Part 2 can be used for the calcium oxide determination. It should preferably be carried out on an aliquot part of the nitric acid extract of the concrete to be employed for the chloride determination so that these two determinations are made on the same test portion of concrete and sampling errors are reduced.

However carefully chemical analyses of concrete samples for chloride and cement contents are carried out inherent errors occur at different stages of the analyses. Any errors in the actual analytical determinations of chloride and calcium oxide in the sample tested should be practically negligible. The major sources of error will be connected with sampling from the mass concrete and with the assumptions required to derive the cement content from the calcium oxide (or soluble silica) determination. Under the most favourable circumstances an overall percentage error of about $\pm 5\%$ can be expected for determinations of cement content and of chloride ion relative to cement. This error may reach $\pm 20\%$ or more depending particularly on the care taken in sampling and the consequent magnitude of sampling errors.

Significant carbonation of the concrete and mortar has been found in some Intergrid and non-Intergrid components and it has been concluded that this factor of the condition of the concrete is likely to become more important as the buildings become older (see Sections 7 and 8). Both concrete and mortar can usefully be checked for carbonation using phenophthalein indicator solution on freshly broken surfaces of the in-situ materials. The technique which has been found to be simple to use during the BRE investigation of Intergrid buildings is described in reference (24).

3 Techniques for determining the condition of embedded prestressing tendons

For pretensioned Intergrid columns, it has been found relatively easy to remove the concrete cover of tendons and secondary reinforcement at locations locally where the concrete is cracked and corrosion of the embedded steel has been confirmed. At locations where there was no cracking, removal of cover has been found to be much more difficult and generally it has only been possible with hand tools to remove cover from very short lengths, eg 50 mm. In these cases, no significant corrosion has been found. In view of the difficulty of restoring the cover to give future protection to tendons it is thought that removal of cover from uncracked locations should be avoided in general. An indication of the condition of the embedded steel in uncracked components may be obtained from examination of uncracked sections of cracked components which are being repaired or replaced.

For Intergrid beams with external post-tensioned tendons, visual inspection of most of the lengths of tendons is possible after removal of the mortar cover. Removal of the cover was not found to be difficult where tendons were placed above the top of the flange; it is thought that it would be difficult where tendons have been placed in a channel. This experience has indicated that parts of tendons which are known to be more susceptible to corrosion as described in Section 7 can be checked visually. However, since it has not been possible in the present investigation to 'dissect' a Mark II beam and examine the whole length of tendons it is not known whether other parts of the tendons in these beams may be susceptible to corrosion.

For internally-stressed post-tensioned Intergrid beams, visual inspection of the condition of tendons has been carried out locally by taking cores out of the concrete to the depth of the duct and then removing the side of the duct and the grout with hand tools to reveal the tendons. This technique has been used at several locations along a beam and gives some indication of the tendon condition. It allows also a check to be made of whether the duct is dry and filled with grout at the core locations and samples of grout can be taken for chloride analysis. However, since serious tendon corrosion may occur locally and only a very small proportion of the total tendon length can be examined, the information obtained using this technique should be evaluated with particular caution. The sections of tendon which pass through joints between precast elements of beams are probably less well protected

against corrosion than sections within the precast concrete. In using the coring technique to obtain indications of tendon condition, therefore, some cores should be taken out at the joints.

Examination of inspection techniques used in other fields was concentrated on methods which might be used to check the condition of tendons. Several methods of identifying local corrosion along the length of an embedded tendon were considered:

(1) Measurement of electrical resistance and continuity

The two possibilities examined were the detection of a tendon break by measuring electrical continuity and measurement of area reduction by monitoring increase in resistance to a given current. Both methods were investigated on units in the laboratory and it was concluded that neither can provide a practical means of detecting corrosion in prestressed components. Sufficient continuity was found in most components through the secondary reinforcement, pins, ducts and anchorages to preclude the electrical isolation of any one tendon. For this reason, a break in a tendon would not necessarily cause a break in the electrical circuit and hence would not be detected.

The method of measuring increase in electrical resistance with area reduction was found to be impractical also, because corrosion in the presence of chloride ions tends to be local in nature resulting in a tendon loosing a significant portion of its cross sectional area over only a short length. Changes in resistance would be small therefore and would be reduced even further by the conductivity of the corrosion products.

(2) Use of ultrasonic methods

Consideration was given to ultrasonic techniques based on measurement of either the velocity of sound through components or the time taken for a sound signal to be reflected from a discontinuity in a tendon. Corrosion of steel in concrete would cause changes in both these measurements since corrosion products are less dense than the original metal and a break or severe restriction in a tendon would reflect signals. An appropriate source to produce the required sound energy in the tendons was not found amongst listed manufacturer's products. A second difficulty was the lack of distinction between effects on the measurements due to corrosion and those due to normal imperfections in tendons and their environment. It was concluded that ultrasonic methods and equipment have not yet been developed to provide a practical and useful field technique for detecting breaks or severe corrosion of prestressing tendons.

(3) Use of radiographic techniques

Radiographic techniques have been used successfully to detect breaks in prestressing tendons, voids in the grouting of post-tensioning ducts or layout of reinforcement in concrete. It is possible to detect quite small changes in density either in the tendon profile or the grout, but considerable experience is needed to interpret radiographs correctly. From examination of radiographs taken of prestressing ducts which were subsequently opened for inspection of the condition of the tendons, it was concluded that the technique is not suitable for detecting corrosion of prestressing tendons. In addition the need for radiation protection and the cost associated with this specialist technique may make it unsuitable for general use.

It was concluded that there is, at present, no technique available for checking for the presence of severe corrosion along the whole length of tendons in situ. Existing techniques are limited to visual inspection of short lengths of tendon.

Table 2 Comparison of chloride contents determined by different methods

| Concrete | % Chloride ion by weight of concrete | | |
	by 'Volhard' method (Clause 9.1 of BS1881: Pt 6)	by 'Quantab' method (BRE IS 12/77)	by 'Hach' method (BRE IS 13/77)
a	0.02	<0.03	<0.03
b	0.04	0.07	0.05
c	0.07	0.08	0.09
d	0.13	0.15	0.15
e	0.24	0.23	
f	0.43	0.43	0.44
g	0.46		0.51

10 Survey of overseas experience

A postal survey was made to assess European experience with pretensioned or post-tensioned prestressed concrete. It revealed that some European countries restrict the chloride content of concrete containing prestressing steel to very low levels while still permitting the use of calcium chloride with normal reinforced concrete. In Austria, Germany, Holland, Portugal, France, Luxembourg, Sweden, Denmark, USSR, Czechoslovakia and Hungary the use of calcium chloride in prestressed concrete is prohibited. Such cases of damage which have occurred are due to the unauthorised use of the chemical or incidental use of chloride-bearing aggregate.

The Austrian Standard 'ONORM' B 3233 limits the water soluble chloride content to not more than 0.02% chloride ion by weight of concrete. Chloride content of aggregates is limited to 0.01% chloride ion by 'ONORM' B3304, while the chloride ion content of the mix water is restricted by 'ONORM' B3305 to 1500 mg/litre. Chloride-bearing admixtures for frost resistance are not permitted in reinforced or prestressed concrete ('ONORM' B3332). Where permitted, admixtures may contain chloride but the chloride content of the concrete is limited to 0.002% chloride ion by the weight of cement.

Despite these restrictions certain problems of corrosion of prestressing steel in concrete containing chloride have occurred overseas. In the USSR, for example, prestressed concrete units failed in a concrete factory after 5 months service while in a second case, prestressed concrete units failed 8 months after manufacture and 6.5 months after installation: in both instances high chloride contents were found in the concrete[25, 26].

It was reported from one country that calcium chloride had been used in amounts in excess of 2.0% chloride ion in prestressed concrete units which had led to a loss of bond, cracking and spalling of the concrete cover, fracture or complete corrosion of prestressing tendons. Prestressed components, some near the sea, generally made with good but not homogeneous concrete and containing between 1.6% and 4.0% chloride ion by weight of cement, had produced sufficient corrosion of secondary reinforcement or tendons to cause cracking and spalling of the concrete cover. In several instances failure of prestressed joists was reported.

In Germany, codes and standards limit the permissible chloride content in concrete. For cement (DIN 1164) the chloride is limited to a maximum of 0.1% chloride ion, although typical cement analyses give a chloride content much lower than this. The chloride level when admixtures are used for rapid hardening of concrete (DIN 4226) is limited to a maximum of 0.002% chloride ion by weight of the cement. Limits for the chloride ion content of mix water for prestressed concrete is set at 600 mg/litre. The chloride ion content for mix water used for grouting is restricted to 300 mg/litre. Such strict limits are in use today but it is quite possible that by accident (or design) some chloride will have been added to the concrete of existing buildings. Consequently, programmes for evaluating the effect of chlorides on prestressing steel in concrete have been established in Germany.

These programmes have shown that corrosion damage may occur at low levels of chloride in a wide range of exposure conditions. It should be noted however, that the prestressing steel largely employed in Germany is quenched and tempered which has a completely different metallurgical structure from British cold-drawn and patented prestressing wire and is thereby more susceptible to pitting corrosion and stress corrosion cracking[27].

Calcium chloride has been used as an accelerator for concrete in Sweden. A 1960 report concludes[28]:

(1)   There is no evidence that normal addition of chloride ion to reinforced concrete, ie 0.6% to 1.0%, has caused any increase of corrosion of embedded steel.

(2)   In the cases where addition of calcium chloride could be regarded as the major cause of corrosion, the addition was very large, approximately 2.5% to 5.0% chloride ion.

(3)   Dangerous corrosion of embedded steel has also occurred where there has been no calcium chloride. The main reason was excessive porosity in the concrete or insufficient cover of reinforcement.'

Gukild[29] reports that 'in view of the sensitivity to corrosion of prestressing steel, chloride or constituents containing chloride should not be used in concrete for prestressed concrete bridges.'

Denmark had discouraged or prohibited the use of calcium chloride admixtures.

While the use of chlorides in prestressed concrete is not permitted in the Netherlands, problems have occurred recently with a precast reinforced concrete flooring system[30]. This flooring system consisted of prefabricated 50 mm thick reinforced concrete planks, 2.5 m in width, supported on walls or columns. Above the flooring planks, reinforced concrete, 120 mm to 140 mm thick, was cast in situ. Calcium chloride was found to have been used in the manufacture of the prefabricated flooring units. Widely varying amounts of chloride were found in the concrete, within the range 0.14% to 1.69% chloride ion by weight of the cement. In the investigation, if the measured amount of chloride ion was not more than 0.05%, it was assumed that no chloride containing admixture had been used. The majority of floor panels were used indoors but occasionally some were found externally and had corroded more extensively.

The Dutch working party concluded that at a chloride content of 0.14% chloride ion, the chloride concentration in the pore water in the concrete would be equal to that in seawater. Since bare steel in seawater corrodes at a rate of $60\,\mu$ m per annum it was argued that the durability of reinforcement in a carbonated concrete containing this level of chloride would be unacceptably low compared to the normal life of the building.

To minimise the rate of carbonation and the availability of oxygen to the steel, the report recommends effective sealing of the surface if the chloride level was between 0.1% and 0.2% chloride ion for units used indoors and showing visible rust stains and 0.1% and 0.45% chloride ion for those units with no visible signs of damage. Pitting corrosion of the reinforcing steel was observed at chloride levels corresponding to 0.4% chloride ion and hence the report sets a boundary limit from which progressive corrosion must be assumed. This limit was 0.25% chloride ion for panels showing corrosion and 0.5% chloride ion for those units without rust staining. The summarised boundary conditions for internal and external exposure are given in Tables 3 and 4.

Previously, the Netherlands Committee for Concrete Research published in 1971 the results of a worldwide survey on 'Cases of Damage due to Corrosion of Prestressing Steel'[11]. This survey revealed eight cases where chlorides had been used in the grout or where the aggregates or mixing water had become contaminated with chlorides. The report also included several cases of damage where corrosion of tendons had arisen from their exposure to aggressive action in consequence of inadequate protection by the concrete. It is relevant here to mention that amongst the defects associated with these cases of corrosion in the survey were insufficient concrete cover to the steel, inadequate grouting of cables, water being able to reach the steel and the presence of chloride in the concrete or grout. The time that had elapsed before fracture of the steel had ranged from a few weeks up to 38 years.

As a result of still unpublished electrochemical work performed in 1951, the Belgian CEBELCOR[31] recommends that, 'unless other precautions be taken, Portland cement free of any chloride – containing additions be used for structures of prestressed concrete . . .

As a general conclusion it may be said that the majority of countries from which information is available state that no addition of calcium chloride is permitted in

prestressed concrete. However, several countries have had experience of serious damage or failure due to corrosion of tendons in prestressed concrete arising because the protection provided by the concrete has been inadequate to prevent corrosion. In most cases inadequate protection appears to have been a consequence of the presence of substantial amounts of chlorides in the concrete or of the inability of the concrete or grout to prevent aggressive substances in the environment (water, air, chlorides) from reaching the steel.

Table 3 Schedule for floor panels with a pore content higher than 15% used indoors.

Panels showing corrosion stains[1]		Panels showing no corrosion stains	
Amount of chloride ion to cement in wt. %	Measures to be taken	Amount of chloride ion to cement in wt. %	Measures to be taken
≤ 0.05	local repairs	≤ 0.05	none
0.1 to 0.2 inclusive	1 Check if reinforcement is in carbonated concrete. 2a If not carbonated, repair locally and seal the concrete. 2b If carbonated, no longer include the reinforcement in the structural calculations.	0.1 to 0.45 inclusive	1 Check if reinforcement is in carbonated concrete. 2a If not carbonated, seal the concrete. 2b If carbonated, no longer include the reinforcement in the structural calculations.
≥ 0.25	No longer include the reinforcement in the structural calculations.	≥ 0.5	No longer include the reinforcement in the structural calculations.

[1]This means: panels which show damage, ie corrosion stains and/or visible flaking of the concrete cover to the reinforcement.

Table 4 Schedule for floor panels with a pore content higher than 15% used outdoors.

Panels showing corrosion stains[i]		Panels showing no corrosion stains	
Amount of chloride ion to cement in wt. %	Measures to be taken	Amount of chloride ion to cement in wt. %	Measures to be taken
≤ 0.05	Local repairs and sealing of concrete.	≤ 0.05	Seal the concrete.
≥ 0.1	No longer include the reinforcement in the structural calculations.	≥ 0.1	No longer include the reinforcement in the structural calculations.

11 Discussion of findings

The investigation required:
(1) determination of the extent of defects and the amount and distribution of chlorides in precast prestressed Intergrid structures.
(2) determination of the effect of chloride content, building age and environmental conditions on tendon corrosion and its consequences.
(3) structural appraisal of the effects of tendon corrosion.
(4) identification and development of inspection and testing techniques.

The findings will be discussed under these headings:

(1) Extent of defects and the amount and distribution of chlorides in Intergrid structures.

The reports of inspections indicated that most Intergrid buildings had no visible defects associated with corrosion of tendons or reinforcement and that, where visible defects were present they were confined to a small proportion of components. For beams, severe corrosion of tendons was found in one post-tensioned beam subsequent to its failure and rust staining was reported in a few beams at 12 sites and at 10 of these sites, cracking was also reported. At a further four sites, cracking of a few beams was found without reported rust staining. Surface corrosion of the external tendons of post-tensioned beams was reported at four sites. BRE examination of the tendons at five other sites revealed surface corrosion at locations where the tendons are more susceptible to attack and showed that, in the kitchen and shower areas in one building, the corrosion had advanced to produce significant losses of cross-section. For pretensioned columns the incidence of visible defects was greater, two sites having about a quarter of external columns with rust staining, cracking or spalling and 17 sites having a few columns in a similar condition.

Of the 171 sites of Intergrid buildings which were identified, chemical analyses of concrete samples for chloride and cement content were reported from 109 sites. The results indicated that the precast concrete in more than two-thirds of the building contracts has low chloride contents. However two or more samples from beams in 25 contracts were found to contain at least a medium chloride content and for columns 13 contracts also yielded two or more samples with at least a medium chloride content. The majority of these components were manufactured before 1964. Positive indication that calcium chloride was used in the manufacture of components was given in the reported results from beams in nine contracts and from columns in five contracts. The highest chloride contents were found in pretensioned columns, not in post-tensioned

beams. This bias may be expected since in order to increase the rate of production there could be a greater need to accelerate the hardening of concrete in pretensioned components.

Four manufacturers are believed from the evidence to have produced some of the components which gave a positive indication that calcium chloride was added in their manufacture. For the remainder of these components however, the manufacturers could not be identified. Results from components at other sites thought to have been made by the same four manufacturers showed low chloride contents which indicates that these manufacturers used calcium chloride intermittently, ie not in all their production.

The distribution of chloride content between similar components in individual buildings was generally skewed positively (Figures 20 and 21). This suggests that there is probably a substantial amount of concrete in the components containing twice the average chloride content determined from the samples. The maximum chloride content determined within individual components was typically twice the average but exceptionally was as high as 20 times the average, suggesting that in these cases calcium chloride was added in flake form. It follows from consideration of these large variabilities in chloride content and of the other factors which may influence tendon corrosion that inspection of tendons at the sample locations where the highest chloride contents have been found will probably not identify the worst cases of tendon corrosion present in the building.

The large variabilities found between components and within individual components indicate that analyses of single samples (which are necessarily small in size) taken from two or three components in a building will be insufficient to give an indication of the risk of tendon corrosion. The number of components from which single samples are taken needs to be sufficient to allow realistic estimates of the average chloride content and the shape of distribution of chloride contents. This information can then be compared with that found in the present investigation (see Figures 27 and 28) in order to determine whether there is a higher or lower risk of tendon corrosion being present. From this point of view it appears necessary to take samples from a minimum of 10% of components and at least 20 components.

(2) Effect of chloride, building age and environmental conditions

Chloride contents ranging from a trace to above 7% chloride ion by weight of cement have been measured in Intergrid components. While the most severe corrosion of tendons occurred in units having high chloride content, one important finding confirmed by the site investigations was that chloride content alone was not necessarily the sole factor controlling the initiation or the continuance of corrosion. Cement content, permeability of the concrete, the depth to which carbonation had occurred, the exposure conditions and the age of the structure were also factors. Whether corrosion develops or not is determined by the joint action of all these parameters. In the same environment corrosion may be found in different components or over different sections of the same component where local high permeability, with perhaps low cement content, and high depths of carbonation occur. Adjacent parts of the concrete which may have a higher chloride content but lower carbonation may still provide adequate protection to the steel. Initiation of corrosion therefore takes place at sporadic locations in components. When the concrete is cracked as a result of corrosion of the embedded metal or other causes such as crazing or tensile stress, carbonation can readily occur and the chloride concentration in the moisture contained within the crack will have a significant accelerating effect on subsequent local corrosion and also on its lateral spread along the metal surface. Such effects were observed on the most severely affected Intergrid building in which, on an external column, a 10 mm length of tendon had completely corroded below the spalled concrete cover. In this structure, which contained the highest level of chloride found in Intergrid buildings, about one quarter of external

columns were cracked due to corrosion of tendons or secondary reinforcement after 20 years in service.

At medium or high chloride levels in the concrete, corrosion sometimes occurred when the surroundings were alkaline to phenolphthalein. At levels of chloride, around 1.0% chloride ion by weight of cement, localised conditions caused corrosion even when the surroundings remained alkaline but the most likely environment for corrosion to begin and progress, existed when the concrete was carbonated. The depth of carbonation is time dependent so that at chloride contents of 1.0% chloride ion and below, ie medium and low chloride content, corrosion may not become severe until the carbonation front reaches the steel. Furthermore owing to the ready availability of moisture, corrosion may be expected to start and develop to a degree causing visible cracking on externally exposed components before it occurs on internal members which, although subject to condensation, are kept apparently dry.

Currently other BRE research is investigating the performance of reinforcing steel in chloride-bearing concrete. The average chloride content and cracking of the concrete cover for the specimens used in this work, for some groups of similar Intergrid components and for other groups of prestressed or reinforced concrete components in buildings in service are presented in Figure 27 for specimens or components exposed to wet environments and in Figure 28 to apparently-dry

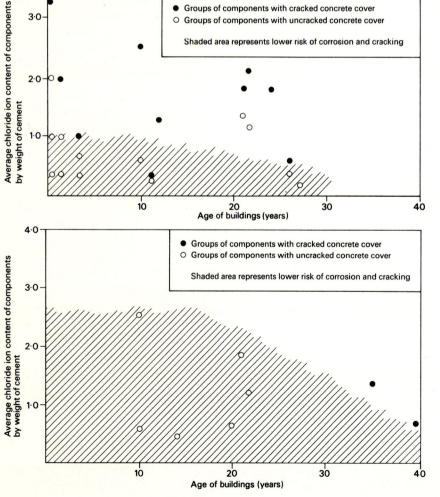

Figure 27 Data from cracked and uncracked concrete components in service in wet, mainly external, environments

Figure 28 Data from cracked and uncracked concrete components in service in apparently dry, internal, environments

environments. The general dependence of corrosion cracking of the concrete on average chloride levels, age and exposure conditions will be seen. No precise boundaries for the areas indicating a lower risk of corrosion and cracking can be drawn but the figures illustrate that corrosion may be progressive under both apparently-dry and wet conditions. The suggestion that corrosion of embedded steel may be progressive in apparently-dry internal conditions is supported by the rust staining and cracking due to corrosion of secondary steel observed in some precast roof components and by the surface corrosion found in some externally-stressed tendons. The figures give some indication of the increase with age in the risks of corrosion and cracking.

(3) Structural appraisal of the effects of tendon corrosion.

An important feature of the tendon corrosion which has been observed in the few Intergrid buildings where deterioration has been found is its local nature. Corrosion has occurred first in those parts of tendons in individual components where the environmental conditions are most aggressive around the tendon and in components subjected to intermittent wetting and drying. Attack has progressed to the stage of severe corrosion of the tendons locally in a few components before corrosion of tendons has developed in all components. The significance of this feature and whether corrosion will be manifest in a visual inspection and of the interplay with the extent of building collapse which may occur on fracture of tendons in one component are the most important considerations relating to building safety. Generally Intergrid buildings appear not to be prone to extensive collapse following a local failure provided that other components in the vicinity of the fracture are in good condition. The sensitivity to extensive collapse will increase if groups of adjacent components become affected by tendon corrosion.

In early Intergrid structures two-way spanning beam grids with external post-tensioned tendons were used for floor and roof structures supported on pretensioned columns. The experience described in Section 6 suggests that cracking, spalling or rust staining will be visible on the faces of columns before column failure occurs. Thus affected columns may be easily identified by careful visual inspection and replacement of affected columns or provision of alternative support can then be considered. Assessment of the two-way spanning Mark II floor and roof beam structures may indicate that there is a capability of transferring the load on a column, should one fail, to adjacent columns. Thus the effects of an individual column failure would remain local in the structure and the building itself would not be in jeopardy. However this mechanism may not protect the building from more extensive collapse if several adjacent columns or adjacent beams in the two-way beam grid itself are weakened significantly by tendon corrosion. For any column the condition of adjacent columns may be manifest by visual inspection

but for the Mark II beam grid it is unlikely that serious corrosion of the tendons in several adjacent beams would be visible in this way. However a proportion of the tendon lengths can be examined visually by removal of the protective mortar as described in Section 9. Such removal at locations where the tendons appear to be most susceptible to corrosion as described in Section 7 will enable inspection of a proportion of the tendon length and thus give an indication of the general condition of tendons. This inspection may assist in judging whether the beam structure has been significantly weakened by tendon corrosion and whether it is, as a result, sensitive to extensive collapse should the tendons fail in one beam or should one column fail suddenly. Corrosion of tendons in several adjacent beams would give cause for concern particularly bearing in mind the proportion of tendon length whose condition cannot be determined.

For beams with internal post-tensioned tendons which were used in some later Intergrid structures, visible evidence of tendon corrosion may not be present before tendon failure. It is possible, however, that rust staining may appear at joints between precast beam elements and visible rust staining and cracking associated with corrosion of secondary reinforcement may give an indication that tendon corrosion is occurring (see Section 7).

In circumstances where evidence, eg visible signs of corrosion and high chloride content, suggests that the condition of internal tendons in post-tensioned beams should be determined small lengths can usually be inspected by coring or drilling the concrete down to the duct as described in Section 9. The condition of the exposed tendons, the presence of voids in the duct and the amounts of chloride in the grout will be factors to take into account in assessing whether severe corrosion is likely to be present in the parts of the tendons between locations of inspection. This assessment will complement the consideration of the probable behaviour of the structure subsequent to a failure of one beam following sudden tendon fracture. The behaviour will be influenced by the amount of fixity at the beam supports and, more importantly in most cases, by the effectiveness of connections laterally between beams, the condition of the structural components, particularly their tendons, and the influence of infill walls and partitions in limiting the extent of collapse.

The BRE investigations have shown that exposure to intermittent wetting and drying increases the susceptibility of components to corrosion of embedded steel. Thus the incidence of corrosion is likely to be greater in components exposed to the weather, eg external columns, or to water leakage. Most roofs of Intergrid buildings are flat and there was evidence at several sites that roofs had leaked from time to time. It appears that roof structures are more likely to be subjected to wetting and drying than in floors and therefore that the risk of tendon corrosion will be greater in roofs. At the same time, ratios of dead load to live load in roofs are higher than in floors so that they are usually 'working' nearer to their design capacity. Consequently, local tendon corrosion is likely to be more critical in roofs particularly also since in some Intergrid Marks there is poorer inter-connection between their beams than between beams in floors. The safety of roofs in Intergrid buildings is therefore more likely to be adversely affected by tendon corrosion than that of floors.

Whilst there are at present no requirements for fire resistance of single storey buildings, the Building Regulations[32] and the Department of Education and Science[33] have requirements ranging from half an hour to one hour for multi-storey buildings depending on the number of storeys. A particular problem relating to fire resistance may arise with Mark II Intergrid buildings in which floor and roof structures are in the form of a grid of beams post-tensioned in two directions by external tendons which were covered by mortar after tensioning. Adequate mortar cover is essential for fire protection purposes where no fire resisting ceiling has been provided or where fire in the ceiling cavity needs to be considered. Inspections in several buildings have shown that the depth of mortar covering on some tendons is very small (see Section 7). Ceilings usually consist of panels mounted on timber or metal strips under the beams but in some cases plaster ceilings are present and in others, eg in some kitchens and boiler rooms, no ceilings are present. The poor cover to tendons and the limited ability of some ceilings to prevent fire reaching the beam structures may result in their fire resistance being less than 30 minutes. Removal of the mortar cover entirely and leaving the tendons uncovered to facilitate future inspections would reduce the fire resistance still further; a fire-proof ceiling would then be essential to increase the fire resistance to an acceptable level. Unfortunately increasing the fire resistance in this way will make future inspection of tendons more difficult and expensive.

4 Identification and development of inspection and testing techniques

Visual inspection has been found to be the best available means of obtaining an early indication of the condition of Intergrid structures. In view of the relationship discussed previously between the time scales of corrosion and a wet or dry environment, particular attention should be given in periodical visual inspections to checking components exposed to moisture and to identifying damp conditions arising from, for example, leaks or condensation. Such checks could provide a practical basis for ensuring that Intergrid structures are kept as dry as possible and hence reduce the risk of premature corrosion.

Visual manifestations of corrosion may be present in post-tensioned beams in the form of cracking or rust staining arising from corrosion of secondary reinforcement, duct liners or tendons. It is clear that the appearance of such signs cannot be relied upon absolutely as a means of detecting tendon corrosion before fracture occurs. However, when they are present investigation of the condition of the tendons would be desirable. Their absence does not prove that the beams have not been weakened by tendon corrosion. Investigation of tendon condition would be necessary in cases where extensive collapse of an important structure, eg a building of large roof span used by the general public, could take place in the event of tendon fracture in one beam, particularly if high chloride contents have been found in the concrete or mortar covering the tendons. Alternatively for these cases action might be taken by modifying the structure to make it insensitive to tendon fracture in one beam.

For pretensioned columns as already mentioned, experience suggests that corrosion of tendons will produce visible cracking, spalling or rust staining of the concrete before remedial measures are necessary. Visual inspection can therefore provide a means of detecting tendon corrosion in pretensioned columns and thus ensuring the columns remain in a safe condition.

Where investigation of the condition of tendons in post-tensioned beams is required available techniques are limited. Visual inspection of short lengths can be carried out after removal of the cover, the inspection of a larger proportion of the total length being possible for external than for internal tendons. Radiographic techniques can be used to determine the presence of tendon fracture or voids in ducts but they are not suitable for general use in detecting the degree of corrosion.

The investigation has indicated the variability that may be found in chloride and cement contents of concrete samples taken from Intergrid buildings. There is variation in the contents between buildings, between similar components within buildings and within individual components. These variations need to be borne in mind when assessing results of tests on samples in relation to the likelihood that tendon corrosion is present and its possible effect on the building.

12 Conclusions

The major conclusions from the investigation of Intergrid buildings are:

(1) From the reports of the inspections at the majority of the 171 Intergrid sites, the structures appeared to be in good condition. Earlier a tendon fracture was found in 1974 in one post-tensioned beam in a non standard Intergrid building which collapsed after 12 years in service and, in these investigations, in one pretensioned column where the concrete was seriously cracked after 20 years in service.

(2) Evidence of deterioration caused by corrosion of tendons or secondary reinforcement was found in about a quarter of column components at two sites and in a few beams at 16 sites and a few column components at 17 sites. Surface corrosion of the external tendons of post-tensioned beams was reported at four sites and found during BRE examination of tendons at five other sites. It had advanced in the kitchen and shower areas at one site producing significant losses of cross-section. There are locations in externally-stressed post-tensioned beams where the tendons are more susceptible to corrosion.

(3) The components in more than two-thirds of buildings for which reports have been received have low chloride contents. The reported results from beams in nine contracts and from columns in five contracts gave a positive indication that calcium chloride was added during manufacture of the components.

(4) Four manufacturers were identified as having sometimes added calcium chloride to the concrete in the manufacture of components prior to 1964. Manufacturers of some components where a positive indication of the use of calcium chloride was obtained could not, however, be identified.

(5) The time scale associated with corrosion of tendons in any prestressed concrete component in service cannot be predicted accurately. In extreme cases severe corrosion of tendons in exposed pretensioned columns of the most seriously affected structures examined had occurred within 20 years; severe corrosion of tendons in a post-tensioned beam indoors, but in a duct partly filled with water occurred after only 12 years. Indoors, in dry conditions, only slight surface corrosion was found.

(6) The chloride content of the surrounding concrete is only one factor in determining the risk of severe corrosion; present data indicate that in external conditions, chloride contents in excess of 1.0% chloride ion by weight of cement present an increasing risk after about 10 years. Nevertheless information from two sites showed that there were a majority of external columns where a high chloride content had not caused visible deterioration after 20 years. Indoors the timescale for deterioration may be much longer. Indoor conditions are usually accepted as being dry but this is not always the case; under conditions which provide free access of moisture (roof leaks, heavy condensation, etc.) the time scale to severe corrosion will be reduced.

(7) The risk of corrosion of embedded steel is determined by the joint action of several factors. Major factors were chloride content of the concrete, age, reduction in alkalinity in the vicinity of the steel associated with permeability and carbonation of the concrete and exposure to moisture. Consequently it is not possible to identify a level of chloride content below which corrosion of tendons in prestressed concrete will not occur in the normally expected building life of, say, 50 years since the action of other factors may lead to corrosion and present experience extends over only 23 years for Intergrid structures. However the risk of progressive corrosion may become significant above 0.4% chloride ion by weight of cement in a relatively short period compared to the intended life of the structure in circumstances where the steel is in an alkaline environment and the concrete exposed to moisture. Indoors the risk appears to be much less than for external exposure except for components in damp locations, eg where there is roof leakage or heavy condensation.

(8) Tendon corrosion usually commenced locally and resulted in a substantial loss of cross-section before the full length became affected. Experience of externally-exposed pretensioned columns indicates that initially severe corrosion of tendons may occur locally in a few components before it develops in all components.

(9) Most Intergrid structures appear to be insensitive to extensive collapse following failure of one component. However some Intergrid structures may be more sensitive than others. The sensitivity to extensive collapse is dependent on the structural design and will be increased if groups of adjacent beam or column components become weakened in the course of time by corrosion of tendons. The safety of roofs is more likely to be adversely affected by tendon corrosion than that of floors.

(10) Periodical visual inspection of Intergrid buildings by an experienced engineer is the best available means, once chloride levels have been established, of obtaining indications of the condition of post-tensioned and pretensioned structures and thus substantially reducing the risk of unexpected failure. In post-tensioned beams the detection of tendon corrosion by visual inspection cannot be relied upon absolutely but it should provide a basis for deciding on the need for further investigation. For pretensioned columns visual inspection will detect corrosion of tendons before serious loss of column strength occurs. During visual inspections for signs of corrosion particular attention should be paid to damp locations. Internally this attention should be directed to roofs, kitchens etc. Corrosion of secondary reinforcement may be indicative of severe corrosion of tendons in both pretensioned and post-tensioned components.

13 Acknowledgements

The investigations described in this report formed part of the research programme of the Building Research Establishment and the report is published by permission of the Director.

The investigations were undertaken by Dr. L. H. Everett and Dr. J. B. Menzies assisted by Mr. R. J. Currie, Mr. W. Lamb, Dr. M. H. Roberts and Mr. K. Treadaway with support of other members of staff in the Organic Materials and Structural Performance Divisions of the Establishment.

Useful advice and assistance was received from representatives of the Building Regulations Division (DOE), the Department of Education and Science, the Property Services Agency, the Scottish Development Department and the Department of Finance (Northern Ireland) who served on the Technical Liaison Committee on Calcium Chloride which was established by the Department of the Environment in April 1977.

Substantial assistance and co-operation was received from many owners of Intergrid buildings and their representatives, particularly from consulting engineers Messrs. Lowe and Rodin, Kenchington Little and Partners, White Young and Partners, W. G. Curtin and Partners and John Nesbit and Partners and from those involved at sites visited by staff of the Establishment. Assistance was also received from the owners of the Intergrid system, Gilbert Ash Limited and from the Transport and Road Research Laboratory, the Cement and Concrete Association and British Rail.

Members of the investigation team wish to thank the many engineers and other people, both in the UK and abroad, who provided so generously much valuable information from their own experience. This help enabled a wider investigation to be made in the short time available and hence conclusions of greater value could be drawn.

14 References

1 Calcium chloride damage in concrete components: Department of Education and Science: 23 December 1976.

2 Intergrid buildings: Department of the Environment/Department of Education and Science, 23 March 1977.

3 **Building Research Establishment.** A simplified method for the detection and determination of chloride in hardened concrete: BRE Information Sheet IS 12/77.

4 **Building Research Establishment.** Determination of chloride and cement content in hardened Portland cement concrete: BRE Information Sheet IS 13/77.

5 Mechanisms of corrosion of steel in concrete: Verbeck G. J.: Corrosion of Metals in Concrete, American Concrete Institute Publication SP–49, 1975, 21–38.

6 **Monfore G. E. and Verbeck G. J.** Corrosion of prestressed wire in concrete: Journal of the American Concrete Institute, 32(5), November 1960, 491–515.

7 **Gjorv O. E.** Control of steel corrosion in concrete sea structures: Corrosion of Metals in Concrete, American Concrete Institute Publication SP–49, 1975, 1–9.

8 **Treadaway K. W. J.** Corrosion in marine environments: Chemistry and Industry, 1976, 348–350.

9 **Roberts M. H.** Effect of calcium chloride on the durability of pre-tensioned wire in prestressed concrete: Magazine of Concrete Research, 14(42), November, 1962, 143–154.

10 **Rehm G.** Damage to prestressed concrete units made with high alumina cement: Zement, Kalk, Gips, No 3, March 1964, 102–111.

11 Cases of damage due to corrosion of prestressing steel: Netherlands Committee for Concrete Research (CUR), Report 49, July 1971.

12 **Lewis D. A.** Some aspects of corrosion of steel in concrete: First International Congress of Metallic Corrosion, London 1961, 275.

13 **Baumel A. and Engell H. J.** Corrosion of steel in concrete: Archiv fur Eisenhuttenwessen, 30, 1959, 417–428.

14 **Hausmann D. A.** Steel corrosion in concrete: Materials Protection, 6, 1967, 19.

15 **Richartz W.** The combining of chloride in the hardening of cement: Zement, Kalk, Gips, 10 October 1969, 447–456.

16 **Blenkinsop J. C.** Effect on normal $\frac{3}{8}$ in reinforcement of calcium chloride additions to dense and porous concretes: Magazine of Concrete Research, 15(43) March 1963, 33–38.

17 **Tomek J. and Vavrin F.** The problem of corrosion of steel in concrete by calcium chloride: Zement, Kalk, Gips, No 3, March 1961, 108–112.

18 **Trudso E.** Corrosion of reinforcement in concrete with calcium chloride: Nordisk Betong, No 4, 1965, 329–346.

19 **Dutron R. and Mommens A.** Corrosion of reinforcement in reinforced concrete: Research Report No 4. Centre National de Recherches Scientifiques et Techniques pour l'Industries Cementière, December 1964.

20 **Gouda V. J. and Monfore G. E.** A rapid method for studying corrosion inhibition of steel in concrete: Portland Cement Association, September 1965, 24–31.

21 **Treadaway K. W. J. and Russell A. D.** Inhibition of the corrosion of steel in concrete: Highways and Public Works, Vol 36 August 1968, 19–21 and September 1968, 40–41.

22 **Gouda V. K. and Halaka W. Y.** Corrosion and corrosion inhibition of reinforcing steel. II Embedded in concrete: British Corrosion Journal, 5(5), 1970, 204–208.

23 **Currie R. J.** The ultimate uncracked shear capacity of low strength high alumina cement prestressed 'X' beams. Building Research Establishment, 1978 (to be published).

24 Carbonation of concrete: Building Research Establishment, 1978 (in preparation).

25 **Krasovskaya G. M.** Reason for the collapse of a precast prestressed truss: Beton i Zheleyobeton, 1969, (4), 20–1.

26 **Alezeev S. N. and Gourovitch E. A.** Caractère de la corrosion de l'armature en fils d'acier à haute résistance de structures précontraintes: Beton i Zheleyobeton, 1967, (6).

27 **Rehm G. and Moll H.** The question of corrosion of steel in concrete: Zement, Kalk, Gips 13(230), 1960.

28 **Bergstrom S. G. and Holst H. B.** The risk of corrosion when calcium chloride is used in concrete: Report 60, Swedish Cement Association, 1960.

29 **Gukild A. I.** Corrosion and protection of concrete structures: Report No 31, Halmstads Jarnverks, 1974.

30 Final Report, Working Group, Monoliet, TNO 1977.

31 **Pourbaix M.** Applications of electrochemistry in corrosion science and practice: Corrosion Science, 14, 1974, 24–82.

Appendix A

Intergrid buildings: Guidance to engineers on visual inspection of precast prestressed concrete and on testing for the presence of chlorides. (March 1977)

Introduction

1. This Guidance Note gives background information on the effects of any calcium chloride present in Intergrid buildings incorporating precast prestressed concrete; describes defects which may be found on visual inspection; and advises on chemical testing for the presence of chlorides.

Background

2. Calcium chloride has been used for many years to accelerate the hardening of concrete, particularly in cold weather. This has been permitted for reinforced concrete with the proviso that the amount should be carefully controlled. In CP 114: 1957, the Code of Practice for reinforced concrete and in CP 116: 1965, the Code of Practice for precast concrete, the limit was set as 2% calcium chloride by weight of the cement. This was on the assumption that the calcium chloride would be in flake form, and the latter code stated that this percentage was equivalent to $1\frac{1}{2}\%$ anhydrous calcium chloride by weight of the cement. CP 110: 1972, the Code of Practice for structural concrete, confirmed this requirement by limiting the total chloride content in reinforced concrete to the equivalent of $1\frac{1}{2}\%$ anhydrous calcium chloride by weight of cement. For prestressed concrete, the Codes of Practice CP 115: 1959 and CP 116: 1965 advised against the use of calcium chloride. CP 110: 1972 recommended that calcium chloride should never be used in pretensioned prestressed concrete, nor in the main concrete of post-tensioned prestressed concrete, unless there was an impermeable and durable barrier, in addition to any grout, between the concrete and the tendons. It also required that admixtures containing chloride should not be used in grouting post-tensioned tendons.

3. The embedded steel in structural concrete is protected against corrosion by the surrounding concrete. The protection depends mainly upon the chemical and physical properties of the concrete (particularly its cement content, degree of carbonation and permeability), the cover to the steel, the degree of exposure of the concrete surfaces and the chloride content of the concrete. Chlorides reduce the ability of the surrounding concrete to protect the steel against corrosion and increase the risk that corrosion will occur. The larger the amount of chloride present the greater are these risks.

4. The effect of excess calcium chloride in reinforced concrete is to cause corrosion of the steel which leads to visible cracking and spalling of the concrete accompanied by rust-staining of the concrete surface. In prestressed concrete, however, visible evidence of corrosion is less likely unless there is secondary reinforcement present. Since prestressing tendons are generally of smaller size than reinforcement in reinforced concrete and are highly stressed corrosion may lead to their fracture and to failure of the component.

5. Investigation of certain Intergrid buildings has shown that calcium chloride has sometimes been introduced into the prestressed concrete and that in some cases serious corrosion damage to tendons has occurred. In one case a post-tensioned beam failed, possibly because the duct liner used was not effective in preventing excessive calcium chloride in the main part of the post-tensioned beams from working through to the tendons.

Visual inspection

6. Transverse or longitudinal cracking or spalling of the concrete may result from corrosion, which may sometimes also be accompanied by rust staining. These defects may become progressively more obvious as corrosion proceeds. All Intergrid prestressed concrete components contain secondary reinforcement: visible evidence of corrosion of this reinforcement indicates that the prestressing tendons may also be corroded.

7. Visible evidence of corrosion in components with pretensioned steel may be limited to cracking as shown, for example, in colour in Plate A1. As corrosion proceeds cracks may widen and lengthen and rust staining may develop (see colour Plate A2). Eventually spalling of the concrete may also occur (see colour Plate A3). The visible evidence illustrated was found to indicate serious corrosion of tendons, significantly decreasing the cross-sectional area of sound steel, and would have led to fracture in a relatively short time.

8. Corrosion in precast components which have external post-tensioned tendons covered by mortar may be indicated by cracking and disruption of the mortar and perhaps rust staining. Where, however, post-tensioned tendons run in grouted ducts or in precast concrete channels filled with concrete cast in situ, corrosion may not be accompanied by such indications.

9. Fracture of pretensioned tendons may not lead to any visible signs additional to those already described, although bowing in columns would usually be expected. Fractured post-tensioned tendons in roofs and floors may be indicated by excessive deflections and possibly by disturbance at the anchorages, separation at the joints in beams of segmental construction or by disturbance of the mortar where beams are externally stressed.

Sampling and analysis of concrete

10. Whether or not there is visible evidence of damage, samples should be taken from the precast concrete and their chloride and cement contents established by chemical analysis. (In the case of beams with externally stressed post-tensioned tendons further useful information may be obtained by testing samples of mortar for chloride and cement content.) This will serve, in cases where visible damage has been detected, to confirm that it was caused by calcium chloride and will be progressive. In other cases it will help in the assessment of the risk of corrosion and future damage. Indeed, it should be recognised that there is a possibility of serious corrosion of tendons not being detected during a visual inspection because the corrosion has produced none of the visible signs described above.

11. Particular care is needed in taking concrete and mortar samples to ensure that tendons are not damaged and that the concrete sections themselves are not unduly affected. The engineer should refer to drawings to determine sampling locations free of embedded tendons and should maintain close supervision during the sampling operation. It will usually be most convenient to take samples by drilling the precast components and collecting the drilled material.

12. There may be considerable variation in the quality of the concrete and the chloride content in any one building. For this reason it will be necessary to take samples of the concrete at several points throughout the structure. It is suggested that the quality and chloride content of the concrete may be assessed by testing samples taken from 10% of beams and columns from each storey. Where there are less than 30 beams or columns in any storey, sampling should take place in at least three beams and three columns. In floors or roofs of grillage construction both primary and secondary beams should be sampled. The components for sampling should be selected at random. In addition it would be prudent to take samples of concrete from any single beams or columns whose failure would cause collapse of a major part of a floor or roof. For externally stressed beams samples should also be taken from the mortar on 10% of the beams with a minimum of three samples being taken where there are less than 30 beams.

13. Chemical analysis should be made in accordance with BS 1881: Part 6. Consideration could be given to reducing the number of samples analysed for **cement content** if the first three samples taken at random from a batch have cement contents greater than 14%. In these circumstances the remaining samples might be analysed for **chloride content** only and the percentage equivalent anhydrous calcium chloride by weight of the cement calculated assuming a cement content of 14%. A minimum of 10 grams of drilled material is usually needed for analysis for chloride only and 25 grams is needed for analysis for chloride and cement content.

14. It may be assumed that calcium chloride has been added to the concrete if two samples out of those taken show a calcium chloride content of over 0.6% equivalent anhydrous calcium chloride by weight of cement. In the event of an isolated result falling above 0.6% consideration should be given to taking further samples.

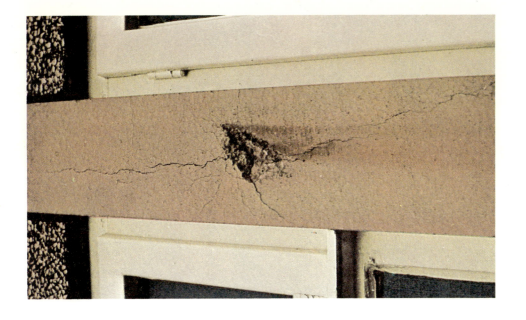

Plate A3 Longitudinally cracked prestressed concrete member with staining and spalling of concrete

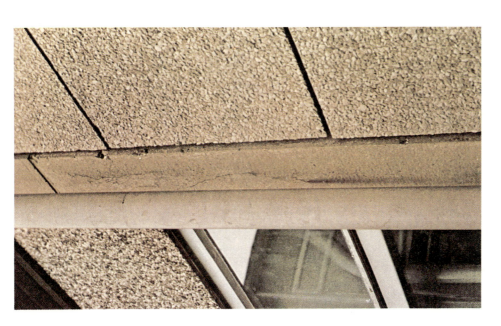

Plate A2 Longitudinally cracked prestressed concrete member accompanied by 'rust' staining

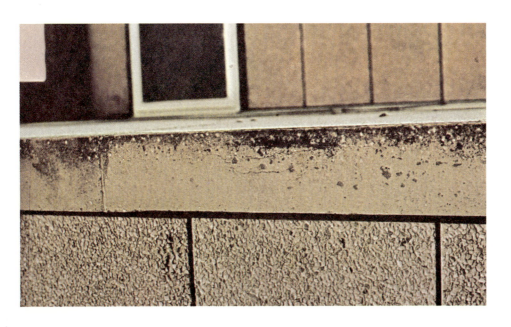

Plate A1 Longitudinally cracked prestressed concrete member

Appendix B

The use of calcium chloride in structural concrete

Chloride salts are present to some extent in most, if not all, structural concretes. This chloride is derived from various sources such as calcium chloride admixtures, sea dredged aggregates, exposure to marine conditions or to chemical de-icing agents. The amount of chloride found in the concrete from such sources may be considerable. Additions of up to 1.5% anhydrous calcium chloride by weight of cement were permitted in the recent past for reinforced concrete while the limit for sea-dredged aggregates was 1.0%, ie 1.0% and 0.6% chloride ion respectively. Amendments to CP 110 have excluded the use of calcium chloride in concrete containing embedded metal and limited the chloride content of reinforced concrete made with marine-dredged aggregates to 0.35% chloride ion by weight of cement for 95% of test results with a maximum limit of 0.5% chloride ion by weight of cement. Uptake of chloride from marine sources and de-icing salts is highly variable but amounts up to 2.5% chloride ion in the surface layers of concrete in bridge decks have been determined. Impurities contained in mixing water, sand, coarse aggregates or in the cement used in concrete also contribute to the chloride content. The amount of chloride obtained from such impurities is usually small; for example, typically the mix water may contain up to 100 mg/litre chloride ion (in potable water) which, with a water/cement ratio of 0.45, would give only 0.005% chloride ion by weight of cement. British cements can contain up to 0.02% chloride ion although the British Standard for Portland cement, BS 12, unlike the German Standard (DIN 1164 which permits up to 0.1% chloride ion), does not prescribe a limit for chloride content. The amount of chloride in quarried aggregates can range from zero to 0.01% chloride ion, the highest chloride content reported to the Building Research Station. While higher chloride contents in the concrete may occasionally occur from such natural sources, the normal 'background' level has been assumed to be below 0.06% chloride ion by weight of cement in CP 110: 1977. Chemical analysis giving much greater chloride contents than this in inland areas indicates that chloride-containing aggregates or admixtures have been used in the preparation of the concrete.

Calcium chloride has been used for many years to accelerate the hardening of concrete, particularly in cold weather, and when permitted, the amount has been carefully specified. The chemical is available, to BS 3587, in flake or hydrated form containing about 25% by weight of water of crystallization. The water content can vary, hence CP 110: 1972 required that the chloride content be specified as the amount of anhydrous calcium chloride, i.e. material containing no water. Earlier Codes of Practice referred to the use of flake calcium chloride (70% to 75% anhydrous calcium chloride). When this solid hydrated calcium chloride was incorporated directly into the mix a very uneven distribution of chloride in the concrete sometimes resulted. Later recommendations indicated that the admixture should be dissolved in the mix water and this method was recommended in the Code of Practice for the structural use of precast concrete, CP 116: 1965. Calcium chloride was also obtainable in liquid form, containing 35% to 37% equivalent anhydrous calcium chloride by weight in aqueous solution. Some cements were produced with integrally ground calcium chloride containing from 1.9% to 2.6% of the anhydrous chemical. Such extra rapid hardening cements are no longer produced and when in production the manufacturers did not recommend their use in reinforced concrete.

The Code of Practice for the structural use of normal reinforced concrete in buildings, CP 114: 1948 in Clause 501(f) referred to work in cold weather.

It stated:

> 'Calcium chloride may be used to accelerate the rate of hardening, usually $1\frac{1}{2}$ per cent by weight of the cement will prove sufficient and there are dangers associated with an excess.'

The reason for the warning was not stated but Scott, Glanville and Thomas [B1] commented:

> '. . . the use of calcium chloride can be of great value for concrete work in cold weather.'

> 'An excessive amount of calcium chloride may cause too rapid setting, leading to difficulty in placing the concrete and may also result in corrosion of the reinforcement. A limit of 2 per cent of calcium chloride by weight of the cement should not be exceeded.'

In the First Report on Prestressed concrete [B2], published by the Institution of Structural Engineers in 1951, it was stated:

> 'Particularly in pretensioned systems, early hardening of the concrete is desirable. A rapid hardening cement should thus normally be used. When, however, an accelerator such as calcium chloride is used in the mix, care should be taken to avoid the risk of initial set occurring inconveniently soon.'

There was no suggestion in this Report that use should be confined to cold weather conditions.

In 1957 Clause 501(f) in the Code was amended to read:

'Calcium chloride may be used to accelerate the rate of hardening of Portland cement concrete but not more than 2 per cent by weight of the cement should be used.'

The comment in the Revised Explanatory Handbook[B3] was left unchanged.

It was not until 1959 in the Code of Practice for the structural use of prestressed concrete, CP 115, that advice was given against its use, specifically to avoid corrosion in prestressed concrete. The following was included in Clause 501(g) and 501(j):

'Calcium chloride should not be used when steam curing is employed.'

'Until more is known regarding corrosion, the use of calcium chloride or salt cannot be recommended. There may be dangers associated with an excess.'

The commentary on this Code by Walley and Bate[B4] contained the following statements:

'The use of calcium chloride in concrete subjected to steam-curing helps to offset the loss of strength at greater ages which would otherwise be experienced with respect to concrete cured normally. Experimental evidence shows that it should not be used in steam cured units with pretensioned steel as it causes corrosion of the steel even when used in proportions not exceeding 2 per cent of the weight of the cement. In post-tensioning, where the tendon is remote from the concrete and may be surrounded by grout free of calcium chloride, the objection to its use might not be as great but as yet insufficient is known of its effect in these circumstances to justify its use.'

'Until more is known of its effect on the corrosion of prestressing steel, calcium chloride cannot be recommended for concreting in cold weather.'

During the late 1950's and early 1960's the Building Research Establishment had research programmes on calcium chloride in concrete. A conclusion of tests on tendons in concrete for periods of up to two years including external exposures,[9] was:

'The present results indicate that with good concrete practice in mix design, depth of cover and specification of materials, the additional corrosion produced by the use of commercial flake calcium chloride up to about 2 per cent by weight of cement in dense, normally cured Portland cement concrete will have no structural significance.'

From tests on reinforcement in concrete under external exposure of up to five years,[16] one conclusion was:

'From the results of this experiment it can be concluded that the use of 2 per cent of flake calcium chloride by weight of cement in a dense, well compacted concrete will have little effect on the degree of corrosion of the reinforcement. In a porous or badly compacted concrete the effect of the calcium chloride is to increase the amount of corrosion which would normally have taken place in the absence of calcium chloride.'

The results of research at that time did not therefore discourage the use of calcium chloride but the Code of Practice for the structural use of precast concrete, CP 116: 1965, was more specific than previous Codes in stating that it should not be used in prestressed concrete. It did however permit its use in reinforced concrete. The recommendations contained the following clauses:

'Calcium chloride should be hydrated calcium chloride complying with BS 3587 and should preferably be in flake form; the total amount present in the concrete should not exceed 2 per cent by weight of the cement. As the hydrated form contains about 25 per cent water, this quantity is equivalent to $1\frac{1}{2}$ per cent by weight of anhydrous calcium chloride. The calcium chloride should be dissolved in some of the mixing water before being added to the concrete.'

'Many admixtures contain calcium chloride, and the Engineer should enquire from the manufacturer of any other admixture he approves for use whether it contains calcium chloride and, if so, the percentage by weight expressed as anhydrous calcium chloride. The amount of admixture to be used should be such that the amount of calcium chloride does not exceed the above limit. He should also enquire whether the admixture will accelerate the setting of the concrete, as does calcium chloride, because special precautions may be necessary to ensure that the concrete can be placed and compacted fully in the time available; under no circumstances should the concrete be 'retempered' by adding further mixing water.'

'Where calcium chloride is used in concrete, not less than 25 mm of cover should be given to all steel unless permanent protection is provided.'

'Calcium chloride is not recommended either as an admixture or integrally mixed with the cement in any form of prestressed concrete work with either pretensioned or post-tensioned steel. It should never be used in prestressed concrete which is to be subjected to curing at elevated temperatures or which will be subsequently exposed to warm, moist conditions. When reinforced concrete is to be steam cured, the addition of calcium chloride is undesirable. Calcium chloride should not be used in concrete made with sulphate-resisting cement.'

Further research at the Building Research Establishment was reported in 1971 which concluded that durability of prestressed steel in concrete would be achieved with the use of dense, impervious and uniform concrete free of chloride and adequate depth of cover to the steel.[B5]

In the following year the Code of Practice for the structural use of concrete, CP 110, 1972 was published. It referred to chloride in Clauses 6.2.2.3 and 6.2.4.2 as follows:

'Marine aggregates may be used provided that the content of chloride salt in the aggregate, expressed as the equivalent anhydrous calcium chloride percentage by weight of the cement to be used in the concrete, does not exceed 1.0%, but where the proportion exceeds 0.1% by weight of cement, marine aggregates must not be used with high alumina cement or for prestressed concrete in circumstances where calcium chloride admixtures are not permitted. In addition, in concrete containing embedded metal, calcium chloride must not be added in such proportion that the total anhydrous calcium chloride in the admixture, plus the equivalent value of anhydrous calcium chloride calculated from the chloride in the aggregate, exceeds 1.5% by weight of the cement.'

'For concrete containing embedded metal the anhydrous calcium chloride content should never exceed 1.5% by weight of the cement and therefore extra-rapid hardening cements should not be used. Where marine aggregates are used the provisions of 6.2.2.3 apply.'

'Calcium chloride should never be used in pretensioned prestressed concrete, nor in the main concrete of post-tensioned prestressed concrete, unless there is an impermeable and durable barrier, in addition to any grout, between the main concrete and the tendons. Calcium chloride should never be used with high alumina cement, sulphate-resisting Portland cement nor super-sulphated cement (see also 6.11.6.3).'

'Whenever calcium chloride is included in concrete containing embedded metal there is an increased risk of corrosion of the metal. It is therefore important that calcium chloride, either in the flake or solid form or present in an admixture is dissolved and thoroughly mixed so as to minimise variations in the chloride concentration throughout the concrete.'

'The corrosion risk is increased still further when concrete containing calcium chloride and embedded metal is cured at elevated temperatures, or is subsequently exposed to warm moist conditions (see 6.11.6.3).'

'It is essential that the mix should have an adequate cement content and a low water/cement ratio compatible with the production of a workable mix so that full compaction can be obtained. Accurate measurement of all the mix constituents, particularly the cement and the calcium chloride, is most important, and the concrete should be thoroughly cured.'

It is perhaps significant that when the Code, CP 110, refers to concreting in cold weather (6.11.7) there is no reference to the use of calcium chloride. Recommendations for grouting cable ducts (6.12.2) contain the following:

'Admixtures should be used only when experience has shown that their use improves the quality of the grout. They should contain no chloride, nitrate, sulphides or sulphites. When aluminium powder is used the total expansion should not exceed 10%.'

In dealing with accelerated curing Clause 6.11.6.3 states:

'Concrete containing embedded metal and calcium chloride should not be cured above 60°C.'

The Handbook[B6] explaining the content of the clauses in CP 110 contains the following statement:

'Calcium chloride. Calcium chloride is one of the most useful admixtures, as it can be of considerable benefit, when correctly used, in winter building, in emergency repair work and in enabling a quick turn-round of formwork. It is, however, liable to lead to some detrimental effects in the hardened concrete particularly if mis-used.'

'The code therefore concentrates on giving details of the maximum permitted dosage of calcium chloride and the method of including it in the concrete, and lists those situations in which calcium chloride should not, or must not, be used. These Code recommendations are extremely important and must be carefully followed if the risk of steel corrosion or excessive drying shrinkage of the concrete is to be avoided. Many admixtures contain calcium chloride and so the engineer must know what the proportion is in order to comply with these limitations. It should be noted that the Code does not permit the use of calcium chloride in reinforced concrete members that are to be cured at temperatures above 60°C.'

The development of these recommendations relating to calcium chloride in Codes of Practice indicate a growing awareness of the potential of chlorides to be a major cause of corrosion of embedded steel in concrete. In 1974 following the collapse of a 12-year-old post-tensioned beam and other corrosion problems in reinforced concrete opinion hardened on the use of calcium chloride in structural concrete and the Property Services Agency prohibited its use. This view was supported by the Cement and Concrete Association and the Building Research Establishment and in 1975 the Institution of Structural Engineers informed the British Standards Institution of their view that the material should not be used in structural concrete. This action led to an amendment to CP 110 which was published in May 1977. It contains the following reference to chlorides in the introduction:

'Over recent years considerable concern has been expressed due to failures in concrete which have been attributed to a number of causes – including excess concentrations of chlorides.

To guard against this, recommendations have been included covering the use of calcium chloride and the limits of chloride in concrete. These clauses are a consensus view reached after considerable discussion within the Committee.

The limit on chloride content in aggregates (particularly those from marine sources) is a matter for continuing research in the light of the present aggregate position in the UK.'

The clauses in the amendment which referred to chlorides were as follows:

'6.2.2.3 Aggregates containing salt or shell. Some aggregates, particularly those from marine and estuarine sources, naturally contain proportions of salts, especially chlorides. These aggregates are suitable for use in structural concrete depending on the type of concrete and total chloride content of the mix (see 6.3.8)

6.2.4.1 General. Admixtures may not be used in 'ordinary structural concrete' by definition (see 6.1.2). Admixtures may be used, however, in 'special structural concrete' but only with the prior approval of the Engineer. Both the amount added and the method of use should be to the approval of the Engineer who should be provided with the following data:

(a) the typical dosage and the detrimental effects, if any, of underdosage and overdosage,
(b) the chemical name(s) of the main active ingredient(s) in the admixture,
(c) whether or not the admixture contains chlorides and, if so, the chloride ion content expressed as a percentage by weight of admixture,
(d) whether or not the admixture leads to the entrainment of air when used at the manufacturer's recommended dosage.

In admixtures for use in:

1) concrete containing prestressing tendons, reinforcement and embedded metal and made with any type of cement, and
2) concrete without embedded metal made with cement to BS 4027 and BS 4248

the chloride ion content should not exceed 2% by weight of the admixture nor 0.03% by weight of the cement.

6.2.4.2 Calcium Chloride. Experience shows that corrosion of prestressing tendons, reinforcement and embedded metal usually results from a combination of factors including excess addition of calcium chloride due to failure to maintain specified dosage, departure from specified mix proportions, poor compaction, inadequate cover and poor detail design.

It is therefore strongly recommended that calcium chloride should never be added to prestressed concrete, reinforced concrete and concrete containing embedded metal.

This recommendation does not apply to concrete which is not prestressed or reinforced or which does not contain embedded metal because there is then no problem of corrosion. In these cases calcium chloride may be used with cement to BS 12 with the prior approval of the Engineer. In specifying the dosage and manner of adding the calcium chloride, attention should be paid to specialist literature and manufacturer's instruction.

6.3.8 Chloride content. The total chloride content of the concrete mix arising from the aggregate together with that from any admixtures and any other source should not in any circumstances exceed the following limits expressed as a percentage relationship between chloride ion and weight of cement in the mix:

Type or use of concrete	Maximum total chloride content expressed as percentage of chloride ion by weight of cement
Prestressed concrete Structural concrete that is steam cured Concrete for any use made with cement to BS 4027 or BS 4248	0.06
Reinforced concrete made with cement complying with BS 12 Plain concrete made with cement complying with BS 12 and containing embedded metal	0.35 for 95% of test results with no result greater than 0.50

Thus, at the same time as a strong recommendation was made that calcium chloride should never be added in prestressed or reinforced concrete, limits were also introduced on the total chloride contents in these materials which are permitted from all other sources including marine aggregates and admixtures.

References

B1 **Scott W L, Glanville W H and Thomas F G.** Explanatory handbook on the BS Code of Practice for Reinforced Concrete: Concrete Publications Ltd, 1950.

B2 First report on prestressed concrete: Institution of Structural Engineers, London 1951.

B3 **Scott W L, Glanville W H and Thomas F G.** Explanatory handbook on the BS Code of Practice for Reinforced Concrete, revised 1957: Concrete Publications Ltd, 1957.

B4 **Walley F and Bate S C C.** A guide to the BS Code of Practice for Prestressed Concrete: Concrete Publications Ltd, 1960

B5 **Treadaway K W J.** Corrosion of prestressed steel wire in concrete: British Corrosion Journal, March 1971.

B6 Handbook on the Unified Code for Structural Concrete (CP 110: 1972), Cement and Concrete Association, 1972.

Printed in England for Her Majesty's Stationery Office by Brown Knight & Truscott Ltd, London & Tonbridge
Dd 586179   K24   4/78